Better Homes & Gardens

diet book

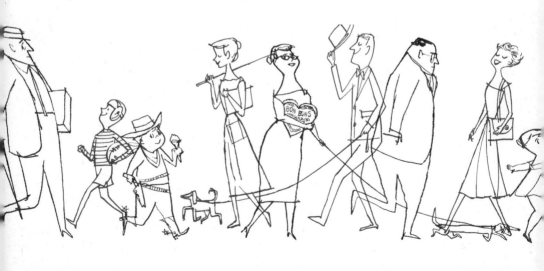

Better Homes & Gardens

diet
book

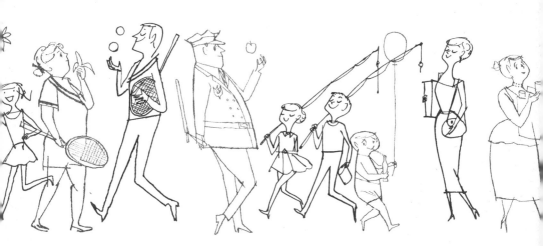

Our happy objective in publishing this new *Better Homes and Gardens* Diet Book is to show people how to eat wisely and well three times a day. Could there be a better reason for publishing a book?

We felt truly fortunate when Donald G. Cooley consented to work with our Foods and Book Editors in developing this book. Mr. Cooley, long a regular contributor of ours, is one of the best informed writers of today on the subject of diet and dieting. As a member of the National Association of Science Writers, he has made countless contributions to science through books and articles.

Dieting demands wisdom and intelligence about nutrition. The meals we suggest were tested in our Tasting Test Kitchen, and they are nutritionally sound as well as resourceful and interesting. They're specifically planned to fit normal family meal requirements.

Better Homes and Gardens reaches over 4,000,000 families every month with new ideas related to home and family. Our purpose and aim has ever been to provide help in finding ways to make life and living a pleasant experience. We publish this new book as a part of this objective, and it is our sincere hope that it will contribute to your health and happiness.

The Editors

The Editors
Better Homes and Gardens

Contents

1 Introduction to good eating   11

2 Do you need to reduce or gain?   15

3 How fat comes and goes   37

4 For safe and sure reducing   65

5 Why proteins are important   75

6 What are your calorie needs?   85

7 *Better Homes & Gardens* meal plans   97

8 When you're away from home plate   147

9 Make use of special foods   155

10 Dieting family style   163

11 What minerals do for you   179

12 If the doctor puts you on a special diet   191

13 Don't overlook calories in alcohol   203

14 All about vitamins   211

15 Cut calories, but enjoy variety   223

16 Your calorie list from A to Z   237

Foreword

The relation of food to health and overweight is of such wide public interest that it has inspired a comparatively large number of books and articles—some good and some bad. Among the latter, the most dangerous are those that are mixtures of truths and half-truths so skillfully blended as to appear honest. Some lack so much in truthfulness that all but the most gullible recognize them immediately as fraudulent. Many write about the good diet in a dull and uninteresting fashion, and even though factual, are heavy and unreadable.

Most welcome, therefore, is a book blending solid facts readably and with a light touch in the telling. And here it is—a book to help you understand clearly how to attain and maintain a good diet.

I contend that the information one must have in order to select a good diet is simple and easy to come by. The accumulated experience of generations has taught us that a variety of wholesome food is essential to all good diets. Variety comes near to being a magic word when you're talking about nutrition.

The good diet includes a variety of fruits and vegetables, of foods from grain and dairy sources, and protein-rich foods such as meats, eggs, poultry, fish, beans, and peas. When the daily menu is made up of some foods from each of these groups, the diet will provide an abundance of essential nutrients for body maintenance and repair, for growth and health.

"Special diets" must be tailored to fit the specific needs of individual people. Therefore, diagnosis is essential before a proper "special diet" can be formulated. This can be done only by a physician. This book repeatedly calls attention to the necessity of professional supervision in all instances which involve disease and therapy.

You who are overweight will find here many guideposts to the slim figure. This book is fun to read, and the information is sound and reliable. Its prime purpose is to see that you use your head more skillfully in the management of your nutritional needs.

James R. Wilson

James R. Wilson, M.D.
Secretary of the
Council on Foods and Nutrition
American Medical Association

Chapter 1

Introduction to

good eating

You ought to like to eat. It's healthy to have a good appetite. It's even better to have one that is wise about foods, trained in the "weigh" it should go. The purpose of this book is to talk with you about how to eat better and enjoy it. The proof of the book is in the eating. We think that there is a lot of good eating in the pages that follow—whether you want to lose weight, or to gain weight, or to feed the family better, or simply to become so well informed about foods that you will forever after feel the utmost confidence in your choices when you scan a restaurant menu or fill your shopping basket.

We believe that the important facts about foods are so simple that any interested person can apply them to his considerable betterment, and that it's nothing against a nourishing meal if it pleases the palate. It must be admitted that some human problems—income taxes and rabbits in the garden for example—can't be solved by diet. But a great many things of vital importance to every one of us are quite directly influenced by what we habitually eat: vigor, growth, disease resistance, appearance, zest, endurance, and even portability.

The modern science of nutrition has discovered so many fascinating things about food elements and the wondrous ways in which our bodies use these ingredients of life, that we propose to discuss the very practical ways in which you can use this knowledge for the improvement of personal and family well-being.

Overweight, which is a polite medical term for too much fat on the frame, is held by competent authorities to be our most serious, chronic, and widespread public health problem. If the urge to be slimmer springs from a yearning to slink instead of slump, to strut instead of waddle, there's no reason to be ashamed of that motive either. It doesn't really matter whether one is motivated by health or beauty.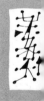

Some overweight persons are not only overnourished but malnourished, if their choices have been self-limited to a few favorite foods that do not supply the variety of elements their bodies need. The *Better Homes & Gardens* reducing diets have been carefully planned, not only to melt off excess fat, but, even more important, to provide nutritive factors that are absolutely indispensable to physical well-being.

You can, of course, plunge right into the reducing diets if you're in a hurry to get going, but we hope you will take a few minutes to peruse the chapters that precede the meal plans. Certain things discussed therein will stand you in good stead for a lifetime, for we assume that you intend to eat all the rest of your life. We will talk about fat, where it comes from, how it comes and goes, who should reduce and why, how to figure reducing speeds, the qualities of wholesome everyday foods that are the keystone of good diets, and sundry other matters that will broaden your background (but not you) and instill confidence in your ability to tell good nutrition from bad.

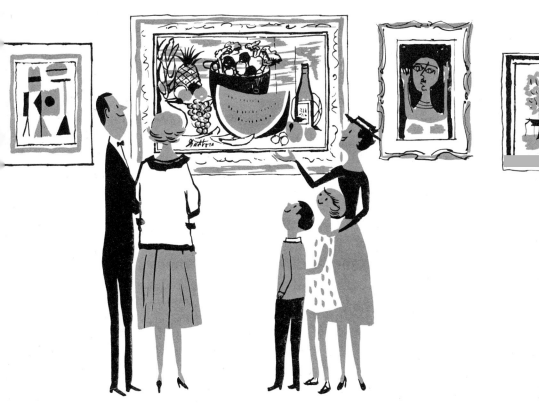

Everyone's interested in food. It's healthy to have a good appetite!

No matter how many diet lists you may have, no matter how much wise and invaluable advice your physician gives about diet, what you actually eat is ultimately a matter of your own choice (unless you're a table captive of someone who prepares your meals), and you naturally want to make that choice as good as it can possibly be. In no other aspect of medicine is control so completely in the patient's own hands as in nutrition. As you read what the experts have to say about various aspects of reducing, you may experience some mild shocks, especially if you've been leaning on a favorite alibi so long it's beginning to bend. But we think you'll agree it's all worth while, when you see the pointer on the bathroom scales beginning to go down, down, down.

Some people do not need to reduce, and definitely shouldn't, but every one of us lives on a diet that is good, bad, or somewhere in between. So we will also talk about the all-important matter of getting more *quality* out of what we eat—packing more nutrition into the children's lunchboxes, keeping proteins, carbohydrates, and fats in healthful balance, choosing wisely when we dine out at restaurants, cafeterias, or corner diners.

A number of charts and tables are included to give quick answers to questions you are going to ask from time to time. The ready-reference calorie table is particularly handy if your physician resents a phone call asking if cabbage has more calories than an artichoke. Speaking of physicians, this book is by no means a substitute for what your doctor will tell you about your individual dietary needs and general state of health.

Chapter 2

Do you need to

reduce or gain

Who says you're too fat or too thin?

You do, probably. Not right out loud, but in those wordless heart-to-mirror talks you have with yourself. Chances are that your opinion is bolstered by remarks of friends, nonfriends, relatives, people you've beaten for office, and others who think they can afford to be frank. Maybe they say it only with their eyes, or little remarks about how size 12 dresses hang on *them* like circus tents until the waistline is taken up. Anyhow, unless you know your weight is just right (in which case you're reading this book to improve the quality of your diet, not the quantity), you have a secret hankering to shed a few pounds or maybe to put on a few.

Your decision that you are overweight or underweight is very likely correct. But you could be wrong, too. It is important to be right, because reducing is not safe unless you have some body fat to get rid of. We mean excess

If you plan to
reduce, get a line
on your weight
from your doctor.

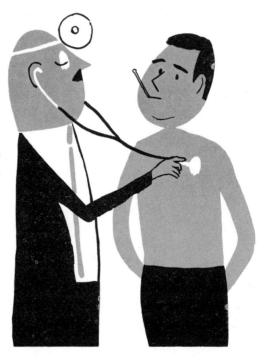

fat, not mere weight. Some sick people are greatly overweight, but not fat at all. They have a disorder which
holds excessive amounts of water in their bodies, and
water is heavy on the scales (it's about two-thirds of your
own weight). Of course, such people need medical attention. Well people cannot use this as an alibi. It's the proportion of fat to the rest of you that is vital, if you plan to
reduce, and the safest way to get a line on your ideal
weight is to have your doctor examine you. If he ap-
proves, go ahead and reduce; if he says no, don't try it.

It's lucky that we don't have to know, down to the last
ounce, what our ideal weight should be. Not even your

doctor can be that precise, unless he weighs you under water. Scales, tables, and your doctor's opinion give all the answers you really need, but you might be interested in some recent research which suggests that our yardsticks of normal weight aren't as exact as they might be.

The gravity of the weight problem

There's a story that Joe Louis caused no end of consternation among doctors who examined him for induction into the U. S. Army. According to height-weight tables, the heavyweight boxing champion of the world was grossly obese, a flabby hulk, a fat man who had to be rejected for overweight. Since Joe was in his prime and about as fat as as a stalk of celery, the doctors couldn't bear to make themselves ridiculous by rejecting him. Conclaves of deep thought were held.

A bright young man suggested that Joe be weighed under water to determine his specific gravity. A fat man floats with ease, for fat is lighter than water, specific gravity 0.93 compared to 1.1 for lean muscle mass. Joe was dunked, and all was well. He wasn't fat after all! He was overweight, but the excess weight came from muscle, not fat. The story may be unauthentic, but the dunking method is used when very accurate estimates of body composition must be made.

Important differences in body weight come from varied proportions of fat (adipose tissue) to lean muscle mass. The range of "normal" body weight is greater than the experts used to suspect, and it is not possible to say,

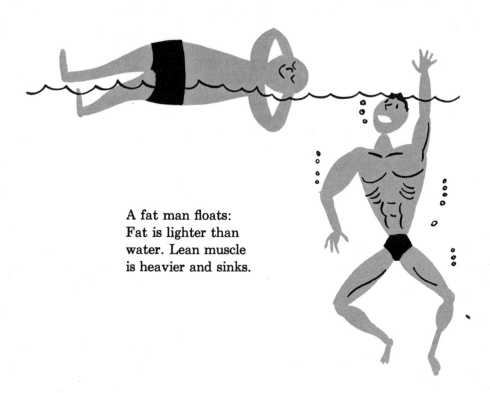

A fat man floats:
Fat is lighter than
water. Lean muscle
is heavier and sinks.

with scientific exactness, where ideal weight for height begins or ends. The lean part of us is more or less constant. It's the part we have to keep feeding generously, or we run into trouble. Excess fat can bury the lean man or woman inside us until it's lost from sight, but it's still there. We can shed excess fat until there isn't any more, and be the better for it.

You're a little different

You and your neighbor can be exactly the same height and weight. But one of you may be fat, the other lean. Dr. R. A. McCance of Cambridge University finds enormous variation of body composition among men and women of normal weight. Captain A. R. Behnke of the Medical Corps of the U. S. Navy analyzed the body composition of 125 sailors, aged 21 to 35. In some of these young men, only 1.5 percent of body weight was fat. In others, fat accounted for as much as 38.5 percent of body weight. Captain Behnke also compared sailors with athletes of the same weight. The sailors had more fat, and correspondingly less muscle, than the athletes. Another study by Josef Brozek compared active and sedentary middle-aged men. The sedentary men had more fat and less muscle than the active ones, although both of the groups weighed the same.

So, if you get a good deal of vigorous physical activity, stair-climbing, golfing, hiking, gardening, and so on, there's a good chance that your frame carries more muscle and less fat than a person of the same weight who lolls in a rocking chair most of the time. Body builds do vary—a perfectly obvious statement, if you take a few minutes to ogle passers-by on a busy street—and some of these differences have applications to diet and nutrition.

The fat, the lean, the muscular

Extreme differences in body build may show up bewilderingly in the same family (Jack Spratt and wife, for instance). Father is a lean, spare fellow who can't put on weight no matter how hard he tries. Mother is plump and chubby and can't get slim. Or the other way around.

You've doubtless recognized different body builds all

your life, without giving them a name. "Sally is just skin and bones," or "Joe has a fist like a pile driver," or "Edna is built like a butterball." For upwards of 20 years, Dr. William H. Sheldon and his colleagues of the Constitution Laboratory, Columbia University, have been photographing and analyzing human physiques (more than 100,000, up to now). Three constitutional factors, in different proportions, seem to enter into the build of all human bodies. Doctor Sheldon has given these factors names that are beginning to become familiar in popular language—ectomorph, mesomorph, and endomorph. You may have heard those names.

To oversimplify it, the extreme ectomorph tends to have a skin-and-bones body build; the mesomorph has big bones and powerful muscles, the endomorph has a superb digestive tract and tends toward roundness and plumpness. We can't possibly be as scientific as Doctor Sheldon, and for present purposes probably shouldn't be, since some folk might use body build as an excuse for doing nothing about diet.

So, with apologies in Doctor Sheldon's direction, we're going to take some liberties with his classifications— partly because you should get some fun out of it, as you observe that people are different and that many of their differences show up at the table. The person who puts on fat with every morsel of food he eats (or so he thinks) has a different diet problem from the lean dyspeptic with whom nothing much agrees and who doesn't agree with anything much. But we hope that the main dividend you will get from our very sketchy discussion of body builds is the realization that good nutrition, eating habits, and figure control are matters of a *lifetime*, not of "going on a diet" for a few days and thereafter reverting to old habits.

The beanpole

Slimness, small bones, slight muscles, an appearance of fragility, generally mark the person who goes through life being called "Skinny" and hating it. Underweight, not overweight, usually is the big problem, and often the very slim person has tried and failed to put on weight by stuffing himself or herself with big, rich meals that the stomach won't tolerate for long. For this extreme of body build—the Jack Spratt type—often has a stomach and digestive tract of small capacity, and perhaps of considerable sensitivity. A little food appeases appetite quickly; a lot of rich food, at one time, overtaxes the capacity and causes misery. Frequent, small meals, distributed through the day, are better suited to "Beanpoles" than one or two big meals spaced far apart. But each small meal should carry a full quota of nutrients.

The plump and the padded

You have met people who can eat practically anything, and do, in large quantities and with every indication of continuous enjoyment. Chances are that they have superb, capacious stomachs and durable digestive tracts that aren't annoyed by rough stuff, bran, coarse fibers, or anything swallowable. Their efficiency as food-stokers (often accompanied by disinclination for vigorous exercise) makes overweight an almost inevitable result unless self-restraint is imposed. In general, the body build tends toward roundness, smooth skin, fat layers beneath the skin so there are no sharp "corners," large thighs and upper arms, but small wrist and ankle bones. A familiar and lovable example: The motherly woman who is a wonderful cook, loves to see kids eat, keeps the cooky jar filled, samples her own cookery in continual kitchen snacks that "don't count"—and worries about overweight. A typical good reducing diet, furnishing lots of satisfying bulk but low in calories, is ideally suited to the plump and the padded.

The big muscle boys (or girls)

These folk may seem overweight according to standard tables, but many are not truly fat. The excess weight comes from heavy bones, powerful muscles, not fat. These men and women love physical activity, are good at athletics and sports, walk vigorously as if the feeling of muscles in use gave them real pleasure. In youth, they may eat hugely but burn up excess calories by excessive activity, and thus do not become fat. But in later years, when energy output slackens somewhat, they may continue to eat as much as when they were younger. This amount, once just right for maintenance, then becomes quite sufficient to lay down fat deposits. These folk usually aren't very finicky about food, are more inter-

Body-build differences
may influence your shape.
You're a bit different.

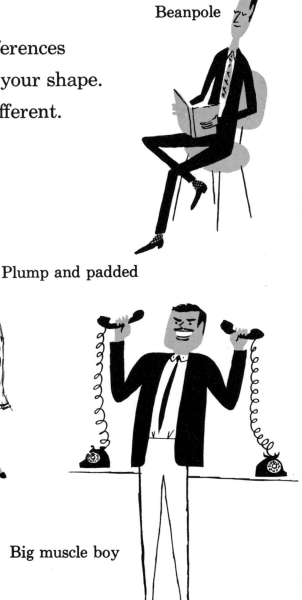

Beanpole

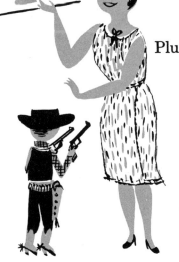

Plump and padded

Big muscle boy

ested in quantity than fanciness, but they should watch for warning signs of "middle-age spread" and cut down on calories as the furious energy expenditure of youth begins to slacken.

You and the weight tables

By now you'll agree that you are a unique person and entitled to be different—well, reasonably different. You will want to know how your weight compares with figures accepted as desirable or average for men and women in general. Before going on a diet to change your weight in any direction, be sure that it should be changed. Ask your doctor first. And find where you weigh in on a reliable height-weight chart, such as the one that follows. As we have said, height-weight tables do not tell you *your* ideal weight to the last half-ounce, but they do tell the awful truth, and sometimes shout it, if you're very far off the beam. The tables on pages 26-29 are reprinted through the courtesy of the Metropolitan Life Insurance Company.

This table is more individualized than many, since it makes some allowances for native differences in body build such as we have been discussing. Don't conclude wistfully that yours is a large frame, unless it is. Heft of bone structure is best judged from size of wrists, ankles, feet, and fingers, where fat isn't likely to mask your framework. A goodly number of fat people actually have small to medium bones and fairly slender wrists and ankles. Extreme beanpoles, of course, have small bones, but fatness is never their problem, except negatively.

One thing sure, if you already weigh less than the figure given for you in the table, don't you dare to reduce without doctor's orders. If you weigh more than the largest figure given for your height, chances are your doctor will say reducing is in order. If your weight is 10 pounds or more in excess, there's very little doubt about what he will say. How he says it depends on his courtliness: "Get rid of that blubber," or "A modest loss of adiposity will make you feel better."

Got a full-length bathroom mirror? A sectional one will do if it reflects the right sections. Shuck your vestments and stand up to the mirror, full-face and profile. Any spare tires or fleshy droops in your reflection? If any-

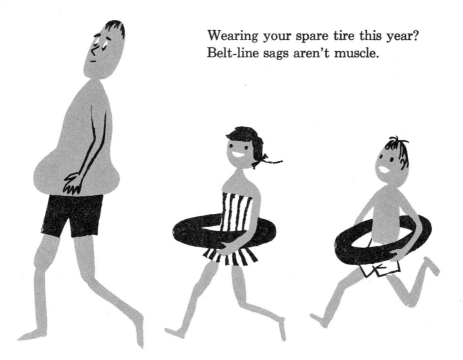

Wearing your spare tire this year? Belt-line sags aren't muscle.

Height and weight
chart for women

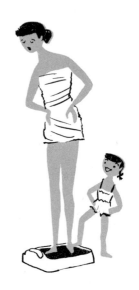

Your bones make a difference in how much you weigh. That's the reason for separate charts: small, medium, and large build. The wide line on our graphs is for leeway. Suppose you have a small frame and are 4'11", any weight from 104 to 111 *could* be your weight.

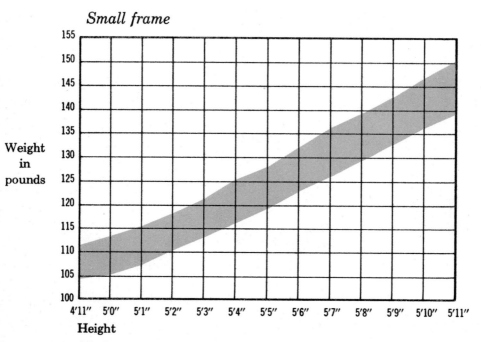

Small frame

Weight in pounds

Height in two-inch heels; weight as ordinarily dressed.

Medium frame

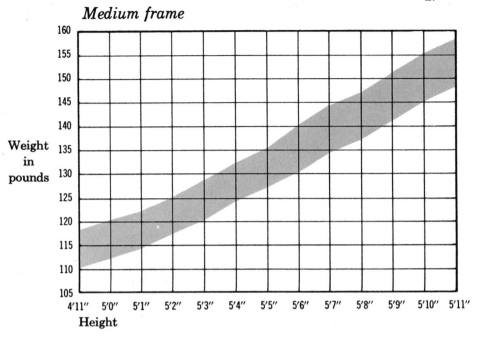

Large frame

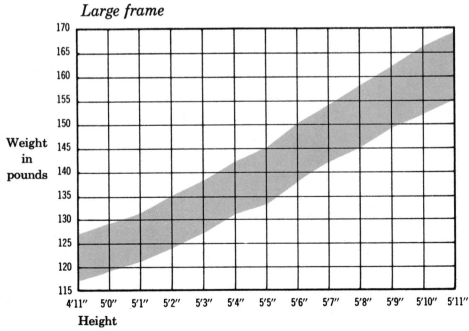

Height and weight
chart for men*

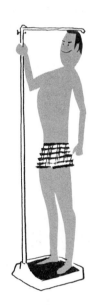

The mere fact that your bones are bigger or smaller than the next fellow's entitles you to weigh more or less than he. By looking at your wrist or ankle bones, decide your category. Your weight should fall somewhere on the pink path as it crosses your height.

Small frame

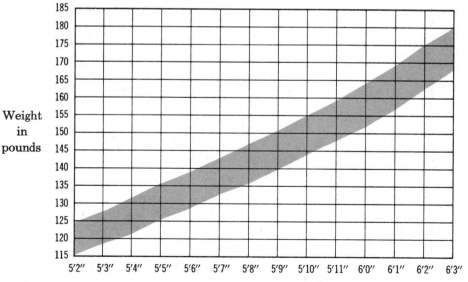

Weight in pounds

Height

Height and weight as ordinarily dressed.

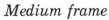

Medium frame

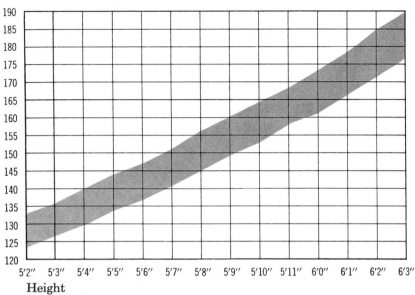

Weight in pounds — Height

Large frame

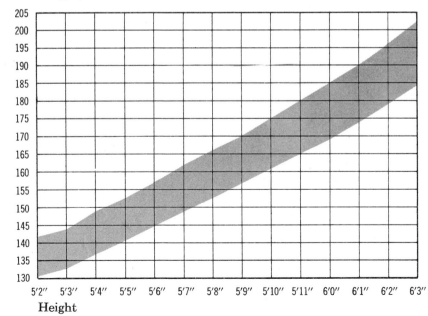

Weight in pounds — Height

thing droops or sags over your belt line, it isn't muscle! Suppose you're a man with legs as lean as a distance runner's. Doesn't mean a thing. Look upward, brother! Favorite areas for fat deposits are a little different for the sexes. Here are the body regions to check:

Women: Fat accumulates under the chin (all of them, if multiple), back of the neck, breast, abdomen, buttocks and hips, thighs, legs above the knees.

Men: Fat accumulates under chin, back of neck, abdomen, trunk.

These are general tendencies of fat distribution, somewhat variable according to amount of fat deposited and other factors. But it's rather common for a man with excess weight to have rather lean legs, lean buttocks, with

If you wonder if

it's really fat,

here are

revealing signs

you can look for

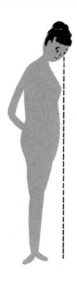

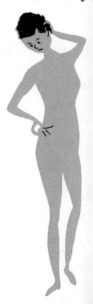

Pinch, ponder. Und
the fat is the real y

Does a protruding
waistline obscure toes?

most of his surplus fat concentrated in a paunchy bay window that may make him lean backward a little to keep his balance when he stands (a spurious kind of good posture). In general, obese women may have slender lower legs but fat concentration between knees and breasts, including the thighs, buttocks, lower back, and that encompassing area of anatomical geography genteelly referred to at the bridge table as "the hips."

Here are some other ways to judge if it's really fat. Stand erect, sink your chin into your chest, gaze down hopefully. You ought to be able to see your toes without a turtlelike extension of the head. Pinch a little flesh, in a suspect area, between thumb and forefinger. If you tense your abdominal muscles, as if a blow were coming your

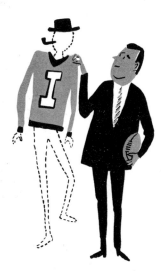

Modeled your college wardrobe recently?

Compare measurements now and 5 years ago.

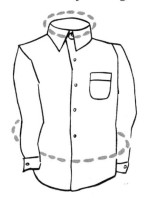

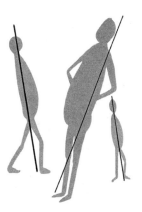

Lean backward to keep your balance?

way, what you'll be able to pinch between thumb and forefinger will mostly be your layer of fat padding. Get the feel of it, reflecting, as you pinch, that the real you lies underneath this layer. We need a little superficial padding, here and there, but if too much of it is here and not enough there, reducing may be in order. Half a century ago, some doctors began to estimate body-fat deposits by pinching skin folds, as we have described, and measuring thickness with calipers. Dr. Ancel Keys of the University of Minnesota recently exhibited a refined pair of calipers for quick and accurate measurements of fat. You can't be that precise. Just pinch and ponder.

Other clues: Have you added a good deal of weight since your mid-twenties? Do your clothes have to be altered frequently to contain you comfortably? What are your waistline, neckline measurements today, compared to 5 or 10 years ago?

Weight through the ages

Weight of a normal or average man or woman is about 15 pounds greater in the forties than in the twenties. We may think that domestic exercises, such as stretching the dollar, make our muscles bigger as time goes on. But too many studies prove that this "normal" increase of weight with age isn't due to inflated muscles or vital cells. It's fat.

And there's more fat than meets the eye. Reduced activity which generally accompanies advancing age brings reduction of cell mass, muscle stuff. So the increased weight of older years is not merely the fat that steps up the poundage, but some extra fat which replaces the shrinkage in cell mass. Of course you and I will never be elderly. An elderly person is always somebody a year or two older than we are. Just the same, we'll be wise to accept our poundage at age 25, say, as pretty close to our ideal weight—a target to shoot at, with your doctor helping to draw a bead on it.

Don't children and adolescents ever get unhealthfully fat before they're 25? They do indeed, and the chubby wallflower at the prom, the lad callously called Fatty by his friends, give a real tug to the heart. Even babies can be too fat, and the Council on Foods and Nutrition of the American Medical Association is concerned about excessive addition of carbohydrates to some infant foods, which do plump up the baby but at some cost to other factors of nutrition. It is especially important that the weight and diet problems of children be worked out in cooperation with the pediatrician or family physician, since this is the time of life when they are building the food habits—good or bad—that may endure through adulthood and into old age.

If you think Jimmy is too thin and ought to be stuffed (with food), or if Susan wants to live on cucumbers because she thinks she's revoltingly convex, see how their weight compares with averages of boys and girls in the following table. Then, if they seem to have too much or too little ballast, ask the doctor. If not, you may be worrying needlessly about skinniness, or you may be letting a teen-ager with weird ideas about an ultraglamorous bean-pole figure put something over on you.

Height and weight
charts for boys

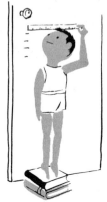

The pink section on chart is "average" zone. Whether your child is at the top of the area or near bottom makes little difference. The height-weight relationship is most important.

Height

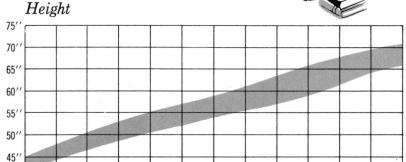

| | 5 yrs. | 6 | 7 | 8 | 9 | 10 | 11 | 12 | 13 | 14 | 15 | 16 | 17 |

(Height axis: 40″ to 75″)

Weight

Weight in pounds

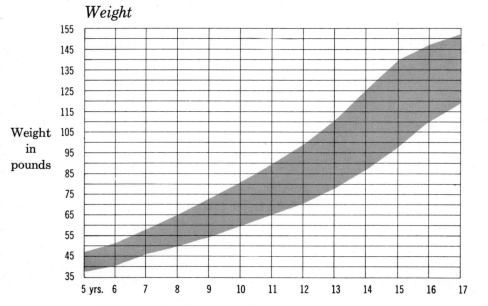

| | 5 yrs. | 6 | 7 | 8 | 9 | 10 | 11 | 12 | 13 | 14 | 15 | 16 | 17 |

(Weight axis: 35 to 155)

Height and weight
charts for *girls*

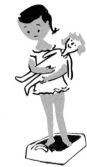

If your child's weight over a period goes up rapidly while height for the period is constant, he is probably gaining too fast. Your doctor will examine and tell you what to do.

Height

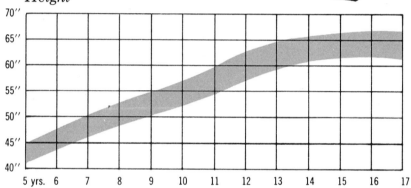

Weight

Weight in pounds

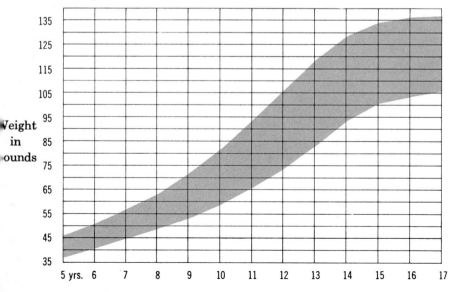

Weight isn't everything

You can be fat, or thin, or just the right weight, and still be malnourished—starved for something you aren't getting. Weight tells a good deal about how much you eat, but practically nothing about quality. You make an unconscious decision about food quality every time you open your mouth to put something into it (except a thermometer). In our country, where food is so abundant that overweight is a grave public health problem, usually it's as easy to pick a good mixture of foodstuffs as an inferior mixture. It feels swell to get rid of excess fat, but don't let the bathroom scales decide whether your diet is good or bad. Before going on any diet, gird yourself with a few simple facts about food. They're quite fascinating, not at all hard to take. And pretty handy to know in this day when food fads, peculiar diets, extraordinary foods and wonderful pills promise astounding miracles to the unwary.

Chapter 3

How your fat

comes and goes

Let's talk bluntly, in a way that loses friends but fat too. By the next paragraph, you may be getting hot under the collar. For we're going to tackle the delicate subject of why some people get fat and some don't. What the experts say may sound boorish, rude, and preposterous to your way of thinking. (A friend who interrupted Bernard Shaw while he was thinking was told, "I'm just rearranging my prejudices.") You'll want to be shown. And you should be tough about making us prove it. Unless you're honestly heart-deep sold on scientific truths that give a pretty rough deal to alibis and short-cut miracles, all is lost except obesity. But if you become convinced, you'll have a wonderful weapon for winning not only the weight battle, but the war. You'll know why a sound reducing diet cannot fail to melt off excess fat, and why better eating habits will keep it melted.

We assume that your weight is greater than your doctor says is good for you. Medical scientists know why you're too fat.

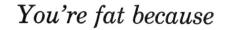

You're fat because

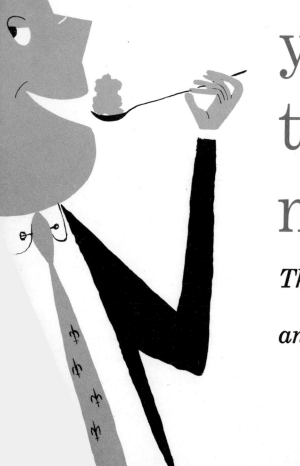

you eat
too
much

There isn't

any other reason

To be sure, there may be a score of reasons *why* you overeat. Psychiatrists, biochemists, and nutritionists have interesting differences of opinion about that. But they're unanimous about one result of overeating: You get fat.

Now we'll have to convince you.

Never underestimate a calorie

This is the way of it: Food furnishes heat energy. It furnishes other things too, and some elements provide little or no heat energy, but a primary fact about food is that it is a fuel. A myriad of complex body furnaces have to be stoked by food. This fuel property is measured in calories. Calories tell how much heat energy is furnished by foods, but they tell nothing else about them.

Every time you expend some physical energy, whether by sawing wood or lifting a skeptical eyebrow, you use up some calories that came from food. In fact, you sleep off several hundred calories every night (and should weigh a trifle less in the morning). While you sleep, your heart beats, you keep on breathing, you radiate heat from your skin. These things use heat energy. Even if you don't move a muscle, do nothing at all, you can't help burning calories as long as you are warm to the touch.

Now, if your meals supply exactly as many calories as you get rid of by bodily activities, if intake equals output, your weight doesn't change. But suppose you consistently eat more calories than you can spend for energy purposes? Where do the extras go? There's no convenient chimney they can escape through. Nature hates waste, anyhow. Surplus calories might come in handy, after you've starved for three days. So they're squeezed into the most compact organic storage unit that nature has invented: fat. This is distributed as charitably as may be on your person.

Body fat is not an inert storage depot, as used to be thought. The fat you have today is not precisely the same fat you had yesterday. Modern studies have proved that fat participates quite busily in endless bodily exchanges. Body fat is like a warehouse that constantly receives new freight consignments, while parcels go out in a steady stream from the shipping room. As long as incoming freight equals outgoing, the warehouse stays filled to capacity, but a lot of business has been transacted. So even if today's fat isn't identical with yesterday's, it's just as much and just as conspicuous.

The moral is that there is only one possible way for fat to get into your body—through your mouth.

Can't we breathe ourselves fat?

We take in oxygen with every breath, and isn't oxygen burned in the body? It is indeed. Don't try to live without it. Then why can't we breathe ourselves fat? Why blame everything on overeating?

Well, hold a lighted match in an empty fireplace and try to warm yourself at the ensuing conflagration. Oxygen of the surrounding air enables the match to burn, but you can't burn a fireplace full of air alone. In the body, we need the latent heat energy of food as a fireplace needs wood or coal. Oxygen is a great little combuster. But there just isn't any way of breathing yourself fat on air alone.

It's a pity, in a way. If farmers could fatten hogs and cattle by turning them out to breathe, giving them nothing to eat, they'd do it in a minute. Where they'd sell their cattle, if we ourselves could get fat on air, is another matter.

So far, we're left with the mouth as the only portal of entry for body fat.

Could your glands be guilty?

There's another theoretical way by which you might get fat without overeating. Suppose that some tricky little mechanism of your body, entirely beyond your control, manufactures fat far and above the call of duty. This engaging idea is quite popular with some overweight folk, for it's quite clear that if this mischievous quirk of metabolism is beyond human control, there's no sense in cutting down on food intake. The supposed cause of this guiltless kind of overweight is identified and lambasted over many a bridge table. It's glands.

Nobody dares deny that glands can be associated with overweight. Or with underweight, diabetes, romance, bulging eyes, or, to wrap it up, the whole business of staying alive. Glands can have very powerful effects on the *distribution* of fat on the body. Some disease conditions are marked by accumulations of body fat so characteristic that a doctor can almost diagnose them at a glance.

Perhaps one or two cases of overweight out of a hundred

may be "glandular." Some clinicians and writers of medical textbooks feel that the glands are the primary cause of obesity in such instances. Many others believe it is a secondary or come-along-for-the-ride cause. Sometimes it's a chicken-or-the-egg problem. Which comes first? If glands can cause obesity, it may be just as possible that overweight can depress the glands. Indeed, infertility

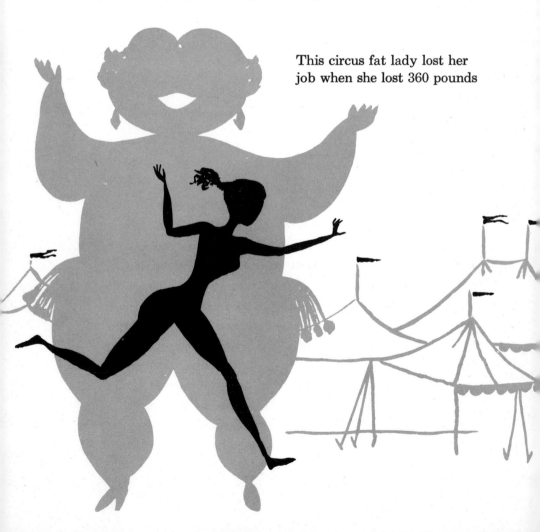

This circus fat lady lost her job when she lost 360 pounds

clinics have many case histories that indicate this is so. Childless, obese wives have succeeded in becoming pregnant with no other treatment than a reducing diet to get rid of excess fat.

But there's another fact which seems to bring in a verdict in favor of those who hold that glands, alone, unfed, all by themselves, cannot cause excess fat. "Glandular" overweights lose body fat, like anybody else, when put on a sufficiently restricted diet. To the extent that glands contribute to fat-making, they need raw materials to work with. Necessary materials come from food. Otherwise, with the right kind of glands, we'd become fatter and fatter while we starved and starved. Nobody can make something out of nothing, except a spouse bent on picking an argument.

Consider the case of a circus Fat Woman who strained the scales at some 500 pounds. Side-show patrons must have muttered sorrowfully about the bad glands that condemned her to a lifetime as a freak. One day the quarter-ton woman began to reduce. When she got through, she weighed 140 pounds—the normal woman who had been inside her all the time. She said she never felt better in her life. True, she lost her job, but she'd been supporting two other women on her shoulders and elsewhere for years, and expenses must have dropped a lot.

Real gland troubles require medical treatment. They can be more immediately serious than even obesity. If an overweight woman sincerely believes that glands make her fat, she should logically rush to her doctor for an immediate checkup. If she doesn't, she probably has a sneaking suspicion that overeating may have something to do with it after all.

"It runs in the family"

And so we come to heredity, the old refrain that "Dad and Mom and my sisters and brothers and aunts and cousins are all fat, so what can I do about it?" Frequently, what is inherited is a good cook or a father who is more than a good provider. Example + opportunity = proficiency in stowing it away. It is possible, and indeed probable, that mysterious differences in body chemistry and psychic make-up lead some people to eat more heartily than others. Many of these subtle differences are doubtless inherited. But the key truth is that we don't inherit fatness per se, and that a sufficiently restricted reducing diet will trim the fat off any obese person regardless of his chromosomes.

Classic examples of hereditary obesity are seen in certain strains of laboratory mice. Unfailingly, generation after generation, these mice become grossly fat, weigh two or three times as much as mice from "normal" families. But that happens only if the fat mice are allowed free access to unrestricted food supplies. They gorge unceasingly, become hopelessly fat, because they never know when to stop eating. Regardless of heredity, the mice can be kept at normal weight by restricting their food. The animals stay slim, but as far as we know are not particularly happy about it.

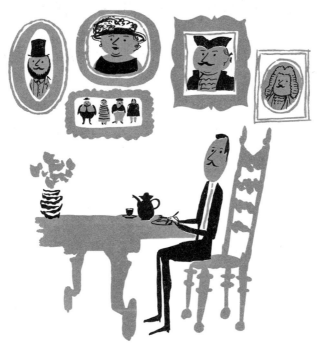

You don't inherit fat—just eating proficiency

There are other ideas as to how people might get fat without overeating. The body might be a super extractor of calories from foods, getting more heat energy out of meals than normal people do. But there's no supporting evidence that withstands rigid scientific scrutiny. More persons than you think apparently believe that drinking water makes one fat. Dr. H. F. Kilander of the School of Education, New York University, questioned thousands of individuals in all walks of life concerning their beliefs about health. Nearly half of them said "water is fattening." It isn't, of course, being bereft of calories. You can drink till you slosh, but that water won't put an ounce of

It won't

rub off

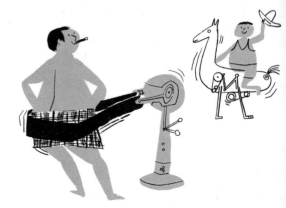

It won't

roll off

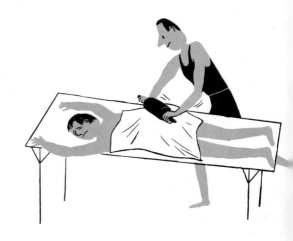

It won't

boil off

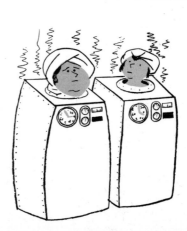

fat on you. True, as long as it's in you, it will register as weight on the scales, but that's a different matter.

The only two ways to reduce

If you've come along with us so far—and you may have been way ahead of us—it is fairly clear that excess fat can be deposited only when more food calories are eaten than the body can burn up for its current energy needs. Intake is greater than outgo, and surplus intake is stored as fat against a lean day. So there are two possible ways in which excess body fat can be gotten rid of.

You can cut down on intake (eat less food).

You can increase outgo (burn more calories, thus making them vanish).

The second of these possibilities is very appealing, because it promises that if you burn up enough calories, you can eat all you want to without gaining weight. You can eat your cake and not have it too. The principle works, too. You can lose weight without ever going on a reducing diet. Although the *principle* is simple, sound, guaranteed to work, its application—at least in the beguilingly effortless forms so often presented to the overweight—can take many tricky twists and turns. Let's see what the experts have to say about it.

It won't rub off, roll off, or boil off

"Increasing the caloric output is extremely difficult and often dangerous." We quote from a report by Dr.

Frank H. Krusen, Chairman of the Council on Physical
Medicine and Rehabilitation of the American Medical
Association, discussing various physical methods that
claim to reduce the fat. You've probably wondered about
the physical methods Council authorities view so dimly.

Hot baths, steam baths, electric-light cabinets, etc. A patient can lose as much as two pounds of weight in an hour
in any kind of hot bath. What's lost is water—sweat—
which is quickly regained from food and drink. Rise in
body temperature can make the system work harder,
theoretically burning up a spare calorie or two. But if you
sat in a bath or cabinet hot enough to give you a 2-degree
"fever" above normal temperature for one hour, you'd
have to take 370 such baths to lose one pound of fat. You
could burn up a slightly greater number of calories by
chewing gum for 370 hours (calorie-free gum, naturally).
Somewhere between those 370 baths you'd probably lose
your gains by eating something. Stimulating cold baths
and needle showers step up metabolism a trifle and increase muscle tone, making many people feel good, but
the calorie loss is about what you get from shivering.

Massage, by hand or mechanical devices. "There is no
scientific proof whatever that massage of any type can be
effective as a reducing measure." It will not reduce local
deposits of fat. It will not increase muscular strength. It
will not cause any significant change in the basal metabolic rate. Harsh words, but that's what the Council's
chairman says. In one famous experiment, laboratory

animals were massaged to see if fat deposits could be
squeezed away or made to migrate. Massage was so vigorous that multiple hemorrhages occurred in the fatty
tissue. But the fat stayed where it was, and in the same
amount; no reduction whatever. Massage has real, important values, but not for reducing—except, some medical observers believe, *after* much fat has been removed
from the entire body by dieting. Then gentle, manual
massage may aid in restoring elasticity to sagging skin.

"Spot reducing." Often, an obese person is less alarmed
by general body weight than by hips, waistline, legs, or
chins that protrude where they shouldn't. They're natural prospects for "spot reducing" gadgets which promise
to flatten the local topography. Chin straps, slimming
creams, reducing belts, rollers, and vibrators are examples. "Mechanical gadgets and 'spot-reducing' appliances are utterly useless for removal of regional accumulations of fat," says Doctor Krusen. "The only effective
way of reducing the fat in local regions of the body is to
follow a program of general reduction of weight by re-
maining on a low-calorie diet."

These methods of removing body weight by increasing caloric output don't seem very rewarding, so far. Can
drugs do a better job?

Drugs in weight reduction

The place of drugs in weight reduction is very simple.
If your doctor prescribes them, take them. If he doesn't,

leave drugs strictly alone. It is true that some drugs can fan body fires into quite a conflagration, burning up quite a few calories, but perhaps some essential parts of you as well. Some years ago, a drug known as dinitro-phenol had a very brief vogue as a weight reducer. It was wonderfully effective in trimming off fat, too. Only trouble was, too many users lost their eyesight.

Today, in the main, there are two drugs which are medically respectable in the control of overweight in certain patients *under a physician's direction*. One of these is thyroid substance.

This vital hormone fans the body's fires to a brighter glow. If the patient's own thyroid gland does not pro-duce enough hormone, supplements can make up for the deficiency. But the surprising fact is that the majority of overweight persons have a basal metabolic rate that is normal or higher than normal, and the wistful hope that fat can be made to vanish safely by merely swallowing a thyroid pill every day is often dashed by the physician.

A second and currently quite popular drug for weight control is amphetamine, in various forms and under various trade names. Capsules may contain vitamins, minerals, bulk-producing substances, and other ingre-dients in addition to amphetamine. The drug postpones sleepiness and fatigue, stimulates mental and physical activity. Thus, as a pepper-upper, it helps to increase energy expenditure. But it also diminishes appetite when taken before meals. And its most important effect is to keep the reducer satisfied with his low-calorie diet. Am-phetamine is always prescribed in conjunction with a reducing diet, never as a capsule allowing you to eat all you want; makes the pangs less disagreeable. Some specialists feel that common humanity justifies the use of appetite-suppressors to tide the patient over the first few weeks of adjustment to a low-calorie diet. Others, just as eminent, advise the patient to scorn the use of props and pacifiers, and to flex his moral muscles while appetite is being re-educated for automatic, lifelong weight control. If taken after noon, amphetamine drugs may keep you awake at night. People are different, and the doctor has to decide about the advisability of drugs in individual cases.

Exercise does burn up calories

There's one way of burning up calories that needs no medical prescription. In fact, if you are holding this book and flipping the pages with your own hands, you're using the method at this moment. It's exercise. We'd like to say that our book reduces you, just by reading it. Could be true, too, if you kept in exact caloric balance and spent an hour a day thumbing these chapters. In another 10 years you might have lost a couple of ounces of fat by faithful reading.

You can see that exercise is a very relative matter, and that its role in weight reduction—a truly important role —needs some understanding if we aren't to be fooled. Some men consume 5,000 to 6,000 calories a day, but never gain weight. They're lumberjacks and other hard physical workers. A fat lumberjack, if he existed, would be fired promptly. The boss-man would know that the fat lumberjack was sitting under a tree instead of chopping. Otherwise, the man would burn up calories like his fellow workers, then he wouldn't be a fat lumberjack.

Theoretically, a person who is many pounds overweight could burn off his fat by exercise without cutting down his food intake in the least. But it's the hard way to reduce. It has been calculated that the average person would have to walk about 36 miles at 3 miles per hour to lose one pound of fat. And we bet you'd be hungry enough, at the end of the thirty-sixth mile, to eat more than you would otherwise.

If it takes so much exercise to shed fat, how is it that football players can lose four or five pounds in a single game? Or that a loss of a couple of pounds is not uncommon after a hot afternoon on a golf course or a vigorous game of handball? Well, most sudden, substantial weight reduction that follows immediately after hard exercise is loss of water (mostly perspiration) that will come right back again.

Nevertheless, the amount of exercise we get during the day, even though it's very little, can make quite a difference in the amount of food we can eat without putting on extra fat. Later, when we give ways of estimating how many calories we need to maintain us each day, we'll see that mild activities can add up—or rather, subtract—a substantial number of calories. Rough, tough, muscle-busting exercise can be dangerous for really overweight people, who already have a heavy burden on the heart and circulatory system.

However, regular, moderate exercise is practically always a very valuable adjunct to a reducing diet, and you will doubtless be so advised by your doctor unless he discovers some peculiar reason why you should never lift a finger. Moderate activity is much better for morale than mooning in an armchair, counting the minutes to the next meal. It's good for general health, tones the muscles, diverts the mind.

Activities you really enjoy are best, because anything that's fun isn't hard work. Walking, swimming, square-dancing, raising Cain, expend various amounts of calories and show you're alive, for you're still moving. You can even ventilate quite a bit of energy driving a car, if there's a back-seat driver along. Any kind of exercise you enjoy is fine if you *stop short of fatigue.* You don't even have to leave home to find activities that are as mild or vigorous as you choose. Spading the garden is hard work, or easy, depending on how long you lean on the handle between shoves. Puttering in a basement workshop, painting a garage, walking behind the boy who mows the lawn to show him the tufts he missed, get rid of a little food energy, and like as not, protect you against temptation. You might become so interested in wrestling begonia tubers that you forget to come in to eat.

Sitting-up exercises (the opposite of sitting down) have their place too. We mean the formal, daily-dozen, swing-squat-kick calisthenics that are done in a routine way. There's one catch. Specific exercises are often taken with the hope that they will reduce one in spots—cause fat to vanish from the hips alone, or the thighs, or the calves, or wherever else the padding is an isolated threat to glamour. Doctor Krusen of the Council on Physical Medicine whom we have already quoted, takes a very scientific and downright stubborn view of this matter. He says that it is impossible for specific exercises to reduce one in certain spots and in those spots alone. To the extent that exercises increase your expenditure of calories, they cause a loss of general body fat. Some of this fat will doubtless be lost from the spots that concern you, but there's no way of removing fat exclusively from a single area, except surgery. This obstinate contention of authorities is not so discouraging as it seems, for it's nice to know that kicking the legs does good for a double chin too.

But local exercises may help to improve one's figure in spots in a different way. Layers of muscle lie beneath surface fat. Fat sags and droops with less restraint when the muscles beneath it are flabby and have poor tone. In extreme cases of obesity, fat may be so thick that muscles are hopelessly outmatched by gravity. But on the whole, exercises that give muscles some fighting spirit are of some aid in restraining bulges, improving posture, and toning up the body so the package is a little neater.

Muscle groups work in pairs: When one member of the team contracts, the opposing member relaxes. Thus each completed motion of an exercise contracts and relaxes all the muscles involved. Different postures and gyrations of formal exercises are merely designed to bring different muscle groups into play. Exercises that require you to swing your arms, kick your legs, or twist your torso are good but, with only your conscience as your guide, may be somewhat less than vigorous. Exercises that make your muscles push and pull against some kind of resistance may make you work harder. Push ups, for instance, compel muscles to work against the resistance of body weight. A simple "bar-bell" prop can be made of a broomstick weighted on each end with a pail containing canned goods. If you are unused to exercises, you will doubtless know what muscle groups you have been using when you wake up the morning after. You can invent exercises of your own, but here are some tried-and-true ones that have stood the test of time:

Modified push-up

Assume the position illustrated, weight on hands and knees, back straight, and head up.

1. Straighten elbows and raise your body off floor. Keep back straight.
2. Bend elbows, resuming original position.

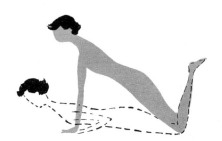

Sit-up

Lie flat on floor, arms extended above head.

1. *Slowly* rise to sitting position. Keep arms extended over head. Bend forward to touch toes with fingers. Keep knees straight.
2. *Slowly* return to original position.

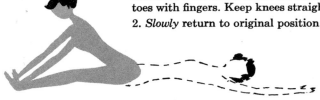

Bicycling

Lie flat on floor, hands on hips. Raise hips, placing weight on elbows.

Make full circles with legs in a pedaling motion.

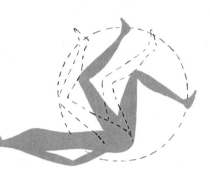

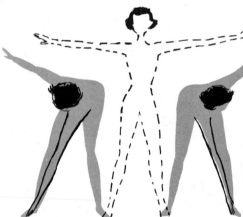

Toe-touching

Stand with feet apart and arms extended sideways at shoulder level.

1. Touch left foot with right arm. Keep knees straight.

2. Return to original position, standing erect.

3. Touch right foot with left arm.

4. Return to original position.

Raising and lowering legs

Lie flat on floor, hands at sides.

1. *Slowly* raise left leg to perpendicular. Keep knee straight.

2. *Slowly* return to position.

3. *Slowly* raise right leg to perpendicular. Keep knee straight.

4. *Slowly* return to position.

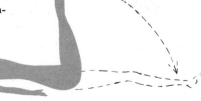

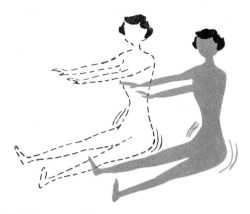

Walking on hips

Sit up straight with arms extended forward at shoulder level, feet apart, knees straight.

1. Shift weight to left hip pulling right hip back.
2. Put weight on right hip shifting left hip back. Repeat 3 or 4 times. Then move forward.

Your own eating yardstick

The reason why increasing one's energy output is hardly ever successful, as a *sole* means of reducing, is that it's brutally hard work. If food intake is unrestricted, relatively enormous doses of physical activity are necessary to get rid of surplus fat.

The easiest way is diet. Would you walk a mile for a coconut cream? You'd have to walk a mile to work off the surplus calories of three coconut creams, and it does seem easier to sit in the sun and not think about coconut creams. Moreover, diet that restricts food intake, while supplying all that is essential, is universally recognized by physicians as the safe and sane way to reduce.

Other measures that help are supplementary to diet. The weight of the evidence is overwhelmingly in favor of *decreasing one's energy intake* (i.e., food energy, calories) as the efficient, healthful way to shed fat.

You may feel that you eat less than certain thin people you know, but they stay slim and you stay plump, and it isn't fair. Some tense, twisty, turbulent thin people waste fabulous amounts of energy. On the other hand, if some overweight persons ate what they say they eat, and honestly think they eat, they'd be mere shadows. Do you really know how much or how little you eat? You and you alone can collect the evidence. We suggest that you keep a daily-diet diary of everything you eat. Don't look up calorie values in the back of the book, yet. Just set down the quantity as accurately as you can.

Fill in the record for a few days, perhaps a week, and don't skip anything you would normally eat because you suddenly feel guilty about it. Then, and not until then, turn to the calorie table on page 237 and add up the answers for the food quantities you have set down. This will give you the approximate daily calorie intake you have been accustomed to. A reducing diet will work just as well for you whether you keep a diet diary or not, but the information you get may be interesting when we discuss the slimming speeds of diets at various caloric levels.

The whys of overeating

If overweight is caused by overeating, the "first cause" of excess fat may be hidden somewhere in the mysterious mechanisms that tell us, "You're awful hungry." Countless people keep their food intake in such perfect and automatic balance with their energy output that their weight scarcely changes. What happens to throw this unconscious regulator out of balance so that those of us who put on weight easily consume more food than we need?

We can't tell you, for the reason that no one factor has been proved guilty in all cases beyond a shadow of a doubt. A great many scientists are trying to smoke out the hunger drive, or the appetite drive, from its hidden lair, which seems to be shaped out of whirling atoms and the lightning dance of molecules engaged in fabulous chemical-making within our bodies. Researchers have identified several factors they believe responsible for excessive food intake, under specified conditions. All are supported by impressive evidence, but no miraculous practical applications. Someday the experts may come up with a pill which balances food and appetite as precisely as the assets and liabilities of a corporation statement, but not yet. We can tell you this: The suspected factors make very handy whipping boys for any overweight person who says "It isn't my fault."

Your old brain. Up near your pituitary gland, about in the middle of your head, nestles your "old brain." Nothing personal: It's old in the scale of human development and was around long before man developed his big broad brow. This area, the hypothalamus, is concerned with regulating body functions we don't have to think about —sleep, temperature, appetite, and such. The central

Daily-diet diary

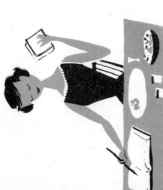

Do you really know how much you eat? To check, keep a diary of *everything* you eat. To check, keep a diary of *everything* you eat. Don't look at calories till the end. Just write in the amounts. Don't skip anything you want to eat because you feel guilty.

	1st day _calorie_	2nd day _calorie_	3rd day _calorie_	4th day _calorie_
Breakfast				
Midmorning snack				
Lunch				
Afternoon break				

Refrigerator raid				
Cooking samples				
Leftovers				
Bridge session				
Munching				
Coffee-klatching				
Party refreshments				
Confections				
Beverages				
Things				
Total				

part of the hypothalamus of animals has been tampered with by scientists, with the most astounding results. Immediately after operation, the animals rush for the nearest food trough and eat voraciously, tripling or quadrupling their weight in an amazingly short time. Eventually, they hit a weight plateau and then eat only enough to maintain their massive weight, but not for very long, as they die prematurely.

Somehow, the damaged hypothalamus sends out false information. It tells the animal it's starving, when it's really suffering from an excess of plenty. Strangely, if certain side parts of the hypothalamus are destroyed, instead of the central section, the effect is just the opposite. The animal loses all interest in food and dies of starvation. Apparently, our "old brain" has something to do with the satiety mechanism that tells us we're full.

Low blood sugar. Quite recent studies from Harvard Medical School suggest that a drive to eat is caused by a fall in the amount of circulating blood sugar (glucose).

It would seem that eating a little ordinary sugar (sucrose) would quickly banish hunger, but it is probably important to use slowly utilized carbohydrate—an apple, banana, slice of bread—to sustain blood-sugar levels for a longer time. Or a protein snack, which has "staying power" and can be converted in part and burned as carbohydrate.

The problem isn't simple, for while some fat and always-hungry animals do have consistently low blood-sugar levels, others, just as fat and just as hungry, have perfectly normal levels. Experimentally, injections of glucose do decrease an animal's food intake, but injections of ordinary sugar or of fat emulsions are without effect. To summarize—there's a lot to be learned yet.

Psychic factors. Some people, when gravely worried, lose their appetites; others smother their worries with food. Specific emotions, then, can hardly be specific causes of overweight, but many clinicians have noted that some patients appear to use food as an escape mechanism for all sorts of frustrations, conflicts, unhappiness, and boredom. But it complicates matters out of all reason to view the average overweight person as a harried refugee from a psychiatrist's couch, a jump or two ahead of the men in white. Some of us like to eat because we like to eat. Who hasn't, on occasion, felt that "Fate cannot touch me; I have dined today"? But knock the "e" out of fate and we've uttered a downright falsehood.

Mysterious chemical factors undoubtedly affect our drive to eat in unknown ways. You smell better—that is, more acutely—when you're hungry. After a meal, even though it's an odorless repast of plain sugar, you aren't so sensitive to scents. Cortisone prods the appetites of many patients.

Two kinds of overweight? Intelligent persons who have put on a little fat gradually, over a period of many years, usually have little difficulty in sticking to a reducing diet if they make up their minds to do so. Often their eating habits are holdovers from younger days, and these habits remain although physical activity which used to burn up calories has lessened. Perhaps they merely stick to the same dietary level they have followed for years, which used to be just right to maintain their weight, but now maintains it with calories left over. If so, it hardly seems necessary to probe into their "old brains," satiety mechanisms, blood sugars, and tribulations, seeking complicated explanations of their table conduct. Other people, who gain weight steadily and rather rapidly, or who have arrived at a plateau where they carry around an alarming excess of fat, may find it difficult to be faithful to a reducing diet. For them, food may have symbolic or special values other than nutrition. A chicken dinner might be a symbol of parental love and happy childhood, when the family sat down to Sunday dinner in the warmth of the old homestead. There may be two kinds of overweight, or even more, reflecting different reasons for overeating. Obesity hasn't yielded all its secrets yet.

Science isn't yet able to say, "This is the one and only reason why people eat too much." As a practical matter, excess fat *always* disappears if food intake is sufficiently restricted, regardless of simple or subtle reasons that lead to overeating. Weight control begins with diet, though it need not end there. Can we prove it? In the next chapter, we'll lay our calories on the table and call for a showdown.

Chapter 4

For safe and
sure reducing

"My husband loves me the way I am. Why should I reduce?" asks an overplump wife. "Sure, I'm too fat, but I feel good, enjoy life, and hate dieting," says an overweight male. Should people who honestly feel that way be bulldozed into reducing? Probably not. A man convinced against his will is of the same displacement still. Reluctant reducers are prone to on-again, off-again dieting, and some lose a couple of hundred pounds a year but wind up weighing about the same as when they started. They fall off the calorie wagon, climb back on again, shed a few pounds, then repeat the cycle, so that their ups and downs in weight, drawn on a graph, look like the scalloped edges of a gingersnap that keep running around the cooky without ever getting anywhere. That kind of oscillating reducing is of doubtful benefit, and it imposes a terrific amount of emotional wear and tear. Also it's only human to become impressed by reasons why reducing isn't a good idea. "It isn't safe," "It leaves me too weak," "Diets just don't work for me."

So if your doctor says you should reduce, it's very important that the reasons why you want to reduce should be felt as deeply in your heart as in your head. Your reasons don't even have to make sense. They can be silly, fantastic, contrary to fact. But if they sustain your faith and determination, they're superior to better reasons that don't really "sell" you. Naturally, it's better if your head agrees with your heart, so we'll fortify you with some 24-carat reasons—but briefly, because we're in a hurry to get on to the luscious pages of good eating that lie ahead.

The high cost of corpulence

Don't be ashamed if the real, secret reason why you want to reduce is to look better. It's a splendid, biologically sensible, socially esteemed reason, and nobody should be shy about admitting it (to oneself). It's healthy for a person to want to look prettier, or handsomer, or downright irresistible. As long as we don't expect a trim figure to bring miraculous blessings all by itself—to win a maid or a man, a salary raise, a coveted job, a movie contract—the drive to improve personal appearance needs no apologizing for.

More practically, the upkeep of a too plump figure is expensive, in other ways than food costs. The joy of picking a smart little number right off the dress racks, at a price that's a steal, is usually limited to women whose figures are fairly standard. And the garment has to under-

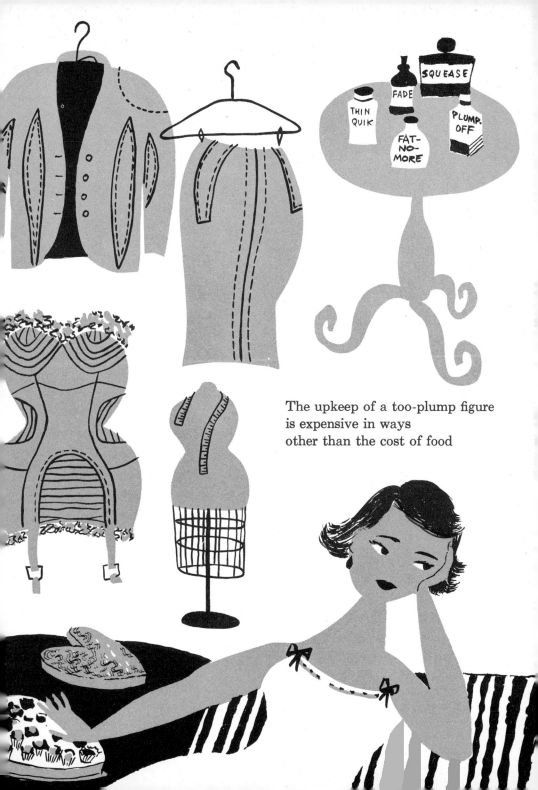

The upkeep of a too-plump figure
is expensive in ways
other than the cost of food

go so many alterations to fit an overweight woman that it's no bargain. Custom-built suits, dresses, girdles, and similar restrainers (don't think that some men don't wear them too!) add to upkeep costs, clothes wear out faster, need cleaning oftener—we don't want to sound like an accountant writing in red ink, but merely suggest that it isn't cheap to stay fat.

It hurts to be hefty

Obesity shortens life. That is the reason why doctors, life insurance companies, and public health authorities are continually urging people to keep their weight reasonably normal. Statistics about the dangers of overweight make scary reading. Of course, statistics do not say anything positive about *individuals*. We can always rationalize that we are exceptions to probabilities that apply to people generally similar to us. We're a little shrewder in making judgments where our personal feelings aren't involved. If you were betting on the outcome of a race between two evenly matched thoroughbreds, one ridden by a 100-pound lad and the other carrying a 300-pound jockey, you wouldn't hesitate long as to which you put your money on.

In just what ways does obesity (which is the same thing as overweight due to excess fat) impair health? Well, it predisposes to, contributes to, or is suspiciously associated with diabetes, high blood pressure, hardening of the arteries, heart failure, gallstones, and gall-bladder disease, shortness of breath on exertion, excessive sweating, flat feet, hernia, degenerative arthritis of hips and knees—let's stop for breath. Nine out of 10 patients who develop diabetes after age 40 come from the ranks of the corpulent. Sustained high blood pressure develops in the overweight at a rate about $2\frac{1}{2}$ times as high as in those of normal weight. Studies at Bellevue Hospital disclosed that hardening deposits in the larger arteries, in advanced stages, were twice as frequent in the obese as in the poorly nourished. Degenerative diseases of the heart, arteries, and kidneys contribute most to extra deaths among overweight persons.

A shocking medical detective story, which might be called *The Case of the Shortened Lifespan*, is told by a study reported by Dr. Louis I. Dublin and H. H. Marks of the Metropolitan Life Insurance Company. Subjects of the study were 26,000 men and 25,000 women who were overweight when they bought insurance policies between 1925 and 1934. They had no other health hazards, but were "rated up," had to pay higher premiums, solely because of overweight. In 1950, the mortality records of these presumably healthy overweight policyholders told this grim story:

Percentage of overweight	Excess deaths above normal expectancy	
	Men	Women
20 *percent*	142 *percent*	139 *percent*
30 *percent*	151 *percent*	148 *percent*
40 *percent*	178 *percent*	156 *percent*
50 *percent*	234 *percent*	175 *percent*
60 *percent* *or more*	282 *percent*	143 *percent*

Women apparently survive excess fat a little better than men (especially when the very fat of both sexes are compared), but in certain overweight-associated diseases, they're more vulnerable than males:

Disease	Excess deaths above normal expectancy	
	Men	Women
Degenerative diseases of heart, arteries, kidneys	149 *percent*	177 *percent*
Gallstones	208 *percent*	284 *percent*
Appendicitis	223 *percent*	147 *percent*
Cirrhosis of the liver	249 *percent*	147 *percent*

In only two categories did the overweight have a better mortality record than standard-risk policyholders. There were fewer deaths from tuberculosis and suicide.

Interestingly enough, the study suggests that overweight is more hazardous at *younger ages.* Overweight men insured in the third decade of life had a mortality rate of 180 percent; fourth decade, 169 percent; fifth decade, 152 percent; sixth decade, 131 percent. A similar trend existed among overweight women. Relative youth apparently does not protect against, but probably intensifies the health hazards of overweight. If we need to reduce, it would seem that the time is now.

Does reducing do any good?

The almost unanimous testimony of those who have reduced is that they feel better, perspire less, don't mind heat so much, get around more spryly, generally get more joy out of life. They get more life from their years, but do they also add more years to their lives?

All the evidence is that they do extend their lifespan. There isn't as much strictly scientific evidence, one way or another, as researchers would like to have, for long-term studies of the benefits of weight reduction are not very numerous. Nevertheless, what evidence we do have is all on the positive side of weight reduction. High blood pressure that often accompanies overweight may subside dramatically when excess fat is shed. Norwegians whose high-fat, high-calorie diet was restricted during wartime had significantly fewer deaths from circulatory diseases.

The life insurance study mentioned before included a number of individuals who were overweight when first examined, but who later reduced their weight sufficiently to obtain policies at standard price or at only a slight added premium. These successful reducers were mostly men (not enough women to be statistically significant). They were divided into classes, according to weight before they reduced: moderately and markedly overweight.

If the moderately overweight men had died at the same rate as men of similar weight who did not reduce, their mortality would have been 142 percent greater than standard. Their actual mortality, after reducing, was only 113 percent. Benefits of reducing were even greater in men who originally had been markedly over-weight. Instead of expected mortality of 179 percent, their actual death rate was down to 109 percent—not very much greater than the normal death expectancy!

This much is certain: If you are overweight and reduce, you have every reason to believe you are prolonging your life, and no reason to think the contrary.

What makes a reducing diet safe?

The most important-if-true reason for not reducing is that it isn't safe, leaves us weak and listless, easy prey for the first sneaky bacterium that comes along. How much truth and how much wishful thinking resides in this idea? The best reducing diet in the world can be dangerous under some circumstances. Faddist diets, weird reducing programs, slimming pills, and so on, can be dangerous under any circumstances. But it is not very difficult to judge whether a reducing diet is safe or wildly wacky. Nor does it require any hidden knowledge known only to men of genius who hug their secrets tightly.

First, as we have seen, *you must have excess fat on your person* for *any* reducing diet to be safe. To slim you, a reducing diet must furnish fewer calories than are necessary to maintain your weight at its present level. Thus you run a calorie deficit, and the calories you need but don't get from your reducing diet are withdrawn from body fat—which is exactly what you want to happen, for the fat slowly disappears. But if there is no surplus fat, the calories you need but don't get will have to be stolen from organs, muscles, tissues, and vital cells. That kind of theft can be deadly. So have your doctor confirm that you are carrying excess fat, before you start reducing.

Second, a sound reducing diet will supply all your

nutritional needs *except* calories. Proteins, vitamins, and minerals, of course. And also many other elements, including those yet to be discovered, which are furnished by common foods eaten in *variety*. A red light, or at least an amber go-slow light, is flashed by any reducing diet that relies largely upon any single food, touted as a "health" food bursting with miracles. All foods are health foods in that they contribute something important to health, but no food is indispensable or indecently miraculous. The keynote of good nutrition is variety of food intake, and will remain so until the experts know more than they do now. As of now, nobody knows enough about the minute chemical needs of the body to concoct a synthetic diet supplying every essential nutrient. But, all these nutrients are contained in the "packages" furnished by three classes of foodstuffs: fats, carbohydrates, and proteins.

Fats and carbohydrates

A tank of fuel oil occupies a lot less space than a pile of cordwood of the same heating value. Fats and oils are just as concentrated sources of heat energy for the body, too. Weight for weight, fats contain more than twice as many calories as carbohydrates or proteins. So fats may be restricted in reducing diets where *reduction* of calorie intake is vital. This can be done safely because, except for vitamin A in butter, margarine, and whole milk, fats and oils do not carry minerals or vitamins or other trace elements along with them, and won't be missed nutritionally. Fats and oils are composed of various fatty acids which may be neccessary for growth and development. Laboratory animals do not thrive if deprived of certain fatty acids for long periods. Not much is known about such needs, but as a practical matter, we're pretty sure to get all the fats we actually require, even on strict reducing diets from which they are presumably barred —green beans and other unlikely foods contain small traces of fat. On normal diets, it is very difficult to obtain as many calories as we need, without eating an impossible amount of bulk, unless fats are used in reasonable to generous amounts. In reducing diets, too, except very strict ones, modest amounts of fat add to that satisfying "filled up" feeling, for fats are slow to leave the stomach.

The bulk of the physical energy of mankind is furnished by carbohydrates—grains, grain products, vegetables, starches, and sugars. Carbohydrate is easily assimilated, is the main foodstuff for muscular activity, and it spares other food elements for other important uses. And, in general, carbohydrate foods supply stomach-filling bulk, generous quotas of vitamins and minerals, and important amounts of protein, at relatively low cost. There are variations in the quality of carbohydrate foods as we actually eat them, for processing and refining may remove some nutrients that were present in the foods in their original state. In normal diets, starches and sugars are very important in satsifying daily calorie needs. In reducing diets, where total calorie intake must be restricted, recommended carbohydrate foods are chosen particularly for their value in furnishing vital elements along with the calories they provide.

Chapter 5

Why proteins
are important

Protein is so famous nowadays, as the indispensable element in safe-and-sure reducing diets, that the word is bandied about pretty glibly. If you aren't too sure just what protein is, don't feel chagrined. It's the most complicated stuff that chemists have to deal with, and they have hardly begun to understand the exciting life processes that depend upon gigantic protein molecules.

Protein is a word of Greek origin, meaning "primal life substance." Before we try to explain what it *is*, you might like to know some of the fabulous things it *does*. To begin with, you are a collection of millions of microscopic cells—a magnificently organized collection, to be sure—and each cell is a fantastic chemical factory which must have protein raw materials upon which its life, and therefore yours, depends. The genes in our cells which give us our heredity, dictate the color of our hair, or its future disappearance, are probably protein molecules.

Muscles, nails, skin, hair, tissues—all of you that's visible and much that isn't—are largely of protein composition. Even your teeth contain minute protein channels (some researchers think that's where decay gets started). It's easy to look into a mirror and reflect that you are gazing upon a superb package of proteins, but chemical activites of proteins you can't see are more astounding.

There are at least 70 proteins in your blood. One blood protein, gamma globulin, is important in giving you immunity to certain diseases. If a measles virus comes along, you "catch" measles. But, stirred to action by the viruses, gamma-globulin molecules change their shapes in such a way as to become antibodies—substances which have exactly the right "fit," so the next time a measles virus comes along, it is effectively neutralized. And you don't get measles twice, well almost never. Your blood contains billions of these tiny protein defenders against various ills. Resistance and immunity to disease depends in part on adequate protein intake.

The hemoglobin molecule that makes your blood red is mostly protein. The "hemo" or iron-containing fraction is a mere 5 percent, and the protein or "globin" fraction is 95 percent. Many cases of simple anemia do not respond to iron tablets alone if underlying protein deficiencies also exist. This explains one way in which stepped-up protein intake may restore zest and vigor to some people who complain of chronic fatigue.

Many hormones are proteins or are intricately assembled from protein elements. And enzymes, those wonderful spark plugs of every single chemical process we live by, are proteins. Sometimes, an apparent vitamin-deficiency disease is not corrected by giving doses of the vitamin alone. Increased protein intake may be necessary before the vitamin is able to do the work it ought to. How can such chemically different things as vitamins and proteins be so dependent on each other? Vitamins are essential parts (co-enzymes) of many enzymes. The rest of the enzyme, and by far the greater part of it, is protein (apo-enzyme). The vitamin is like the sharp, biting tip of an auger that enables the rest of the tool to do its work. Clearly, it is useless to expect vitamins to work miracle cures if a contributing trouble is mild protein starvation.

Children, of course, require more protein than adults (babies, three or four times more, relatively) because they are growing and building *new* tissues. But adults need constantly renewed supplies of protein, too. Wear and tear of tissues requires protein repair. Indeed, the proteins that are you aren't precisely the same as the proteins that were you 10 minutes ago. Studies with radioactive tracer substances prove beyond doubt that proteins of living tissue are constantly being exchanged in a dizzy traffic rush that never ceases for an instant while life remains. Twice a year, you trade in your body for a new one, in the sense that proteins turn over completely in 160 days—even faster trade-ins for your liver, which exchanges its protein in about 10 days.

You get your protein from foods, of course. But foods vary in both the quantity and quality of protein they contain. The differences have to do with little things called amino acids.

What proteins are made of

All proteins are built out of various combinations of 23 different kinds of "chemical bricks." These bricks, or building blocks, are nitrogen-containing substances known as amino acids. How many different combinations (each one a different protein) can be made by rearranging, adding, or subtracting, changing the sequence of 23 structural units? Billions upon billions! The 26 letters of the alphabet spell every word in the dictionary with billions of uninvented words left over.

The proteins you obtain from food are broken down by digestion into the amino-acid building blocks that composed them. In a way, it's as if you swallowed a brick house, knocked the bricks into a loose pile, and then built a new house by picking certain bricks out of the pile and cementing them together. The bricks would be the same ones the original protein house was built of, but the new structure would be as different as a modern ranch house is different from an 1890 mansion. How astounding is the chemical precision of your body, which selects amino-acid "bricks" and builds them into hundreds of unique proteins upon which life processes are utterly dependent!

Your pile of amino-acid bricks, then, had better be good. Although 23 amino acids are known, not all of them have to be obtained regularly from food. But eight amino acids are rated as indispensable. We must regularly obtain these eight from food, and they must be available in the body when they are needed, if we want to stay healthy. Any one of these eight is as essential to good health as vitamins. Animals sicken and die if deprived of just one of these "big eight" aminos. A hormone, an enzyme, a protein necessary for some mysterious body process, can't be made because an essential chemical building block is not on hand at the right time.

So just eating a generous *quantity* of protein foods isn't enough. *Quality* must be there too for buoyant health.

How to judge protein quality

Certain foods furnish proteins that are rated by nutritionists as "biologically complete." They are sometimes simply called complete proteins. This simply means that they furnish *all eight* of the essential amino acids, *all at once*, and in good quantity.

This *simultaneous* need for the indispensable aminos is vastly more important than most of us realize. Experimental work with laboratory animals has piled up some pretty grim evidence. Animals on otherwise adequate diets were given four essential amino acids in the morning. Two or three hours later, they were fed the other four. Thus they received all eight of the indispensable aminos, and in quantities that were more than adequate.

But they died. Amino acids are not stored in the body in any significant amounts. The eight essential ones must be Johnnies-on-the-spot, all present and accounted for, when some essential body protein is in the making. Otherwise, it can't be made. The lapse of a couple of hours between divided feedings of essential amino acids caused the animals to die of subtle protein starvation, although quantity of intake of the elements was abundant.

Although such rigid restriction and division of amino acids practically never occurs in ordinary human diets, wise timing of intake and supplementation of one food by another give very valuable ways of stepping up the protein values of what we eat. A simple, easy-to-remember way of judging protein quality is to think of foods as falling into four general classes:

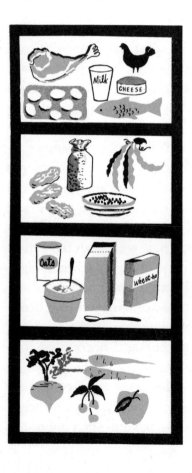

Class 1.
Meat, poultry, fish, eggs, milk and milk products, cheese.

Class 2.
Beans, peas, lentils, peanuts, and other legumes.

Class 3.
Cereals.

Class 4.
Other vegetables and fruits.

Class-1 foods are tops for protein, for they furnish all eight essential amino acids (and others too) at one dose, so to speak. They provide complete proteins. They do not necessarily provide every essential amino in ideal amounts, but there's at least a little of each one, adding up to top quality. Quantity is greatly boosted by aminos provided by other food classes, too.

It's neither necessary nor desirable to live wholly on class-1 foods (nor very thrifty, either). Remember that other food classes supply essential aminos too, but, with rare exceptions that play little part in American diets, single foods of classes 2, 3, and 4 do not furnish them all in one package. Of course, these foods have outstanding virtues of their own and are indispensable for balanced diet, for reasons other than their protein contribution.

And you can make class-2, -3, and -4 foods furnish complete protein—in a practical if not literal sense—by eating a little of some class-1 food along with them. Biologists call it "supplementation." Any essential amino acids that may be missing are furnished by the class-1 food, and the value of the total protein intake is greatly enhanced. Your meal then provides *all at once*—and that is known to be tremendously important—all necessary amino acids, so your body has all the ingredients it needs at the moment to assemble the hundreds of different proteins necessary for health.

A splendid dietary principle is to *eat at least one biologically complete protein at every meal*. This is automatically done if you consume at least a small portion of some class-1 food every time you eat anything at all. Main family meals, usually built around a meat dish, are no problem. It's breakfast, a quick lunch, or between-meal snacks that are likely to be deficient, proteinwise.

A dismaying number of people begin the day with a totally inadequate breakfast. "I'm not hungry," they say. But true physiological hunger should be at its peak at breakfast time, for the body has had no food for eight or ten hours—the longest foodless stretch of the whole day. This may make you suspect that hunger and appetite are two different things, with special significance for reducers. Anyway, for a better breakfast, brimful of bounce, put more milk on your cereal or in your coffee, eat an egg with your toast, or a sliver of ham, or a slice off last night's roast. You get some complete protein which increases the value of fruit juice, toast, and cereal that most of us like for breakfast (don't forget that toast or bread made with dry milk solids contains complete protein furnished by the milk, to enhance that of bread grains). Even on reducing diets, these little protein touches don't rack up an alarming number of calories. Milk can be skim milk; the egg boiled instead of fried.

There are times, of course, when class-1 foods will be skipped from necessity or choice. Then, a wonderful way of improving protein quality is to serve a number of different class-2, -3, and- 4 foods simultaneously, in casseroles and other combinations. Mix them in your meals. Let legumes and cereals and vegetables supplement each other's amino acids. That way, an essential amino acid lacking in wheat may come from a potato. If all this discussion about proteins seems too complicated to bother your head about (you should see how biochemists bother *their* heads!), the main point is that a simple rule of healthful eating has been underscored: Good nutrition is furthered by eating a wide variety of foods, so that the deficiencies of one are made up by virtues of another.

Proteins in reducing diets

It is now pretty clear why so much emphasis is put on protein in reducing diets prescribed by specialists who treat obesity. Reducers, like everybody else, need enough protein, vitamins, and minerals to nourish vital tissues and enter into chemical combinations that keep tissues alive. You could lose weight on a diet limited strictly to whale oil. But for current needs, your body would have to steal little chunks of amino acids from your liver, muscles, or glands, and the real, vital parts of you would starve and waste away.

Adequate protein of sound reducing diets prevents such disasters. Your vital tissues will be just as well fed (probably better fed) as if you gorged on Lucullan repasts from dawn to midnight. You will not be weakened physically. A diet that supplies sufficient protein insures that any loss of weight it brings about is caused by *loss of fat and nothing else.*

Moreover, protein has appetite-satisfying qualities. It stays with you, makes a low-calorie diet easier to take. High-protein foods hardly ever tempt one to overeat prodigiously and therefore to lay on fat. There's a limit to the amount of ground round steak or cottage cheese

84

that one can engulf at a sitting. A person who is truly hungry would as soon eat a pound of cottage cheese as a pound of apple pie. If cottage cheese sounds revolting and apple pie enticing, some factor other than ravenous hunger must be involved. Protein in a reducing diet helps to allay hunger pangs, or appetite pangs, or any reasonable facsimiles.

Another big advantage for reducers is that, generally speaking, protein slims you *faster* than anything else. Foods have a nice, friendly side to them, called "specific dynamic action." In everyday language, foods require that we burn up a few calories to digest and metabolize what we eat. Protein is superior to fat and carbohydrate in this respect. Protein has high specific dynamic action. It fans body fires to a clean, hot flame that keeps a good head of steam in your boiler. This helps to keep human energies at a high level. It also compels us to burn up more calories than we otherwise would.

This speedier-slimming quality of protein, however, applies to protein intake in excess of our basal needs— that is, for repair and rebuilding of worn-out tissue parts, for reconstruction of hormones and enzymes, and so on. Protein in excess of this amount may be burned for fuel, and burned more wastefully than fat or carbohydrate. But this waste, which means wasted calories, is just the ticket for reducers.

So a sound reducing diet furnishes liberal protein for three important reasons: 1. It protects vital tissues from starvation. 2. It is hunger-satisfying. 3. It speeds up the slimming process somewhat.

Chapter 6

What are your
calorie needs?

Slimming speed depends on the ratio between calorie *intake* (food) and calorie *output* (bodily activities). It's a matter of relativity. And the relativity is quite personal, so that a reducing diet of, say, 1,000 calories a day, will not cause fat loss in everybody at precisely the same rate of speed. There are some differences in the way people use and hoard calories that may be unexpected or surprising to you. It helps to know a little about one's own calorific habits, in order to know what may reasonably be expected of reducing diets of various caloric levels.

To begin with, how many calories do you need each day to keep you the way you are? Look up the weight for your height given in the tables on pages 26 through 29. This is close enough to what your normal weight should be. A rough rule of thumb allows 16 calories per pound of body weight for sedentary persons, 20 calories per pound for moderately active persons. Multiply your normal weight by 16 or 20, whichever you honestly feel is most appropriate. The result will be a fair approximation of the daily calories you need to maintain the ideal figure you have or are going to have. Here are recommended daily allowances of the National Research Council:

	Women	Men
Age	(121 pounds)	(143 pounds)
25	2,300 calories	3,200 calories
45	2,100 calories	2,900 calories
65	1,800 calories	2,600 calories

But "sedentary" and "moderately active" are pretty elastic terms. You can get a more accurate estimate of your daily calorie needs if you figure your energy-ex-penditure-per-hour for ordinary activities.

How many hours did you run today? Not as many as you slept. It's fascinating to know that calories are burned while we sleep. You could "sleep off" 1 pound of fat in about 2½ days, providing you didn't wake up to take nourishment. When we're completely relaxed, sleeping, doing nothing at all, not voluntarily moving a muscle, we burn about 1 calorie per minute. This is the fuel needed to sustain basal metabolism. Other activities, from lifting a finger to sawing wood, burn up more calories, in addition to the 1-per-minute for basal needs. Hard physical labor requires us to spend about 4 extra calories per minute, or a total of 5.

Since there are 1,440 minutes in a day (got your pencil out?) there can be enormous range in the calories ac-

How many calories do you burn in 24 hours?

It's easy to overestimate time you spend in vigorous activity. For instance, walking means a brisk pace, not ambling to the water cooler. Put your figures in the spaces around the clock below. Total them at the side. Result is a close estimate of your daily calorie expenditure.

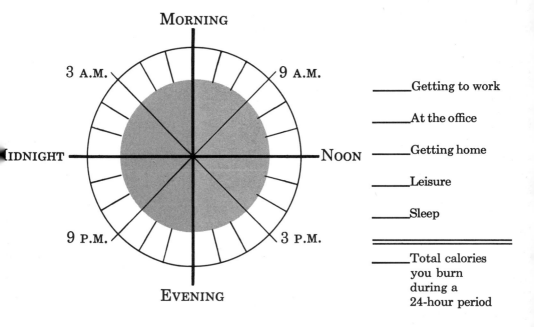

MORNING

3 A.M.   9 A.M.

MIDNIGHT   NOON

9 P.M.   3 P.M.

EVENING

_____Getting to work

_____At the office

_____Getting home

_____Leisure

_____Sleep

_____Total calories
you burn
during a
24-hour period

Estimate your calorie needs from these:

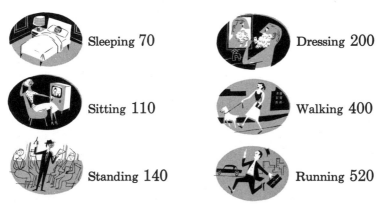

Sleeping 70   Dressing 200

Sitting 110   Walking 400

Standing 140   Running 520

Figures given on this page are based on the average 150-pound male.

tually burned by individuals, according to the time spent doing this or that. And this helps to explain why some people stay fat although they "don't eat enough to keep a sparrow alive."

How sedentary are you?

If you keep a daily-diet diary, as has been suggested, the totals of your accustomed daily intake of calories will tell one of two stories:

1. You may find to your honest surprise that your average daily calorie consumption is greater than you thought —sufficiently greater than the calories you need for maintenance, so that the source of excess fat is obvious.

2. You may find that your calorie intake is not excessive but is just about right for maintenance. In that case, it may seem that you do not deserve to be fat.

The second instance calls for a bit of understanding, for it may lead one to blame obesity upon glands or heredity or some other gross miscarriage of justice. Most people do not continue to put on fat at an excessively fast rate for an indefinite time. Generally there is an initial period of rather rapid and continuous fat accumulation that may last several years. Eventually a weight plateau is arrived at. Food intake is insensibly diminished, to the point where weight is neither gained nor lost to an exceptional degree. At this stage, the patient whose food intake is quite modest may well feel that he does not deserve to be fat. But at some time in the past, he did deserve to be fat, and the ballast lingers on. Some authorities feel that there may be obscure biochemical reasons why obesity sometimes sets in, then settles down, in two-stage fashion, and that if we knew enough about those reasons, weight control would be easier. The practical side of the matter is that a low-calorie diet will remove excess fat no matter how long it has been around.

But it's downright infuriating to discover that someone else, seemingly no more active than we are, stays scandalously slim on a relatively high calorie intake. He eats more and remains slender; we eat less and remain overweight. Let's imagine that two men, or two women, do exactly the same kind of work in an office. They're both sedentary workers, sitting at their desks seven hours a day. But the one who stays slim actually eats more than the one who is overweight. How can that be?

Well, some people are more sedentary than others, although they sit the same number of minutes per day. Overweight induces a certain economy of motion that is quite unconscious. The heavy member of our office pair "sits loose," gives himself up to his chair, muscles blissfully relaxed and perhaps flabby. He reaches leisurely for the phone when it rings, makes fewer trips to the water cooler, is unhurried and unbounceful in everything he does. Altogether, he conserves a surprising amount of energy without appearing to.

The slim one, on the other hand, "fights" his chair, twists, squirms, grabs his pencil tightly, pounds a typewriter as if he were mad at it, and gets out of his chair with a jump instead of an ooze. His muscles are more or less tense all the time, quivering with indignation and

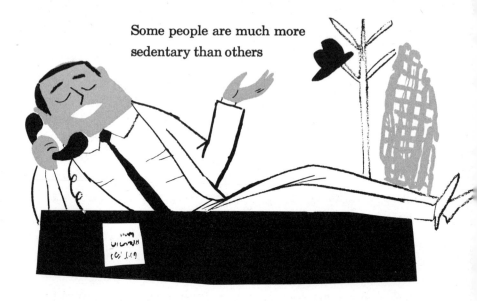

Some people are much more sedentary than others

flipping off calories the while. No wonder he can eat more food without showing it!

If we keep such differences in mind, the consoling idea that overweight is unfair and that excess fat must come unreasonably from nowhere is left with hardly a slim leg to stand on.

Your reducing-diet speedometer

In round figures (what are we saying!), 1 pound of body fat contains 4,000 stored-up calories. The actual calorie count runs a bit less than that, but we want to lean to the conservative side in figuring weight losses, so all your surprises will be pleasant ones.

You now have all the information you need to estimate how fast a given reducing diet will slim you. Here is the formula:

Step 1:

    Maintenance calories minus reducing-diet calories= calorie deficit

Step 2:

$$\frac{4000}{\text{Calorie deficit}} = \text{number of days necessary to lose 1 pound of fat}$$

An example:

Maintenance calories of a
    sedentary, 123-pound woman...2,000
Subtract the calories furnished
    by a reducing diet.............1,500

Daily calorie deficit...............500

4,000 divided by 500 gives 8, the number of days needed to lose 1 pound of body fat. In this example, a

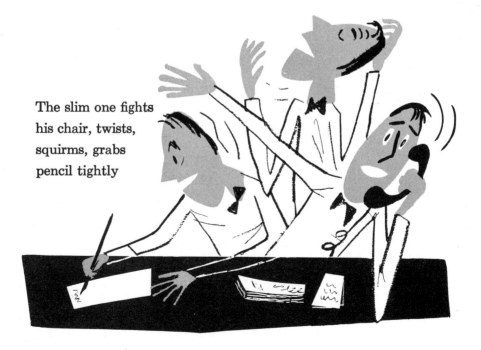

The slim one fights his chair, twists, squirms, grabs pencil tightly

1,000-calorie diet would remove fat twice as fast, 1 pound in four days. Discuss with your doctor the reducing-diet calorie level that is best for you.

It is hardly possible to know *exactly* how many calories you need for maintenance. This need varies from day to day, according to how bustling or lazy you have been. Fortunately, there is one calorie counter that is almost infallible in keeping accounts and telling tales about the shifting relationships between one's intake and output of energy. It's your bathroom scales, the best calorie counter there is. If you do not lose fat at about the predicted rate, the tattle-scales tell one of two stories: Either you've been cheating on your diet, or you have overestimated the number of calories needed for maintenance.

However, there is one important exception to the general infallibility of the calorie-counting scales. It has to do with water retention. Water weighs more than fat, but of course, the water isn't fat. Often, as the body begins to burn fat in making internal adjustments to a reducing diet, there is some temporary retention of water. In fact, for a little while, enough water may be retained so that there is no reduction of *weight* at all, although *fat* is actually being lost.

A very few days—in rare instances, a couple of weeks— bring restored water balance. Then the scales should tell an accurate daily story of *fat* loss—provided one weighs in at the same time of day (preferably on getting up in the morning, after having slept off maybe 500 calories) and not immediately after drinking fluids, which are in the body but not of it.

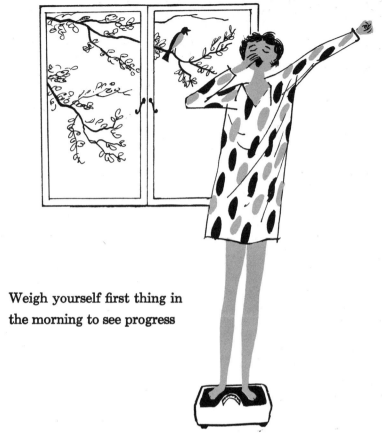

Weigh yourself first thing in
the morning to see progress

On the other hand, many reducers are delighted to find that they lose weight at double speed or even faster during the first days of dieting. If this happens to you, and your diet is twice as good as you hoped it would be, accept the blessing with elation but do not be deceived by it. Much of the extra, surprise-dividend weight loss will be water loss. Don't expect it to continue longer than a couple of weeks. If you do, you will be disappointed later on when your reducing diet seems to have slowed down discouragingly. As a rule, it's easier to lose the first few pounds of fat than the last few, and it helps to remember that fat loss, on a carefully calculated reducing diet, is steady and continuous.

What about "hunger pangs"?

Quite apart from supplying essential nutrients, a sound reducing diet should be *satisfying*. This is accomplished by providing adequate amounts of bulk, sheer stomach-filling substance. Indeed, well-planned reducing diets furnish about as much bulk as average self-selected diets of people who are not reducing.

The importance of bulk for appetite control is perhaps not fully appreciated. We get accustomed to the "feel" of a certain amount of bulk in our stomachs, and if this bulk happens to be less than is customary, we may feel vaguely uneasy and think we are hungry, even though the unsatisfying meal we have eaten may have provided several hundred more calories than usual. During World War II, Drs. R. A. McCance and E. M. Widdowson conducted long-term studies which threw new light on the close relationship of dietary bulk and appetite.

A large number of volunteers lived for three months on a diet that was quite bulky but contained very little fat. "At the close of the experiment," Dr. McCance reported, "four persons who had become accustomed to this food found themselves free to eat what they chose. They continued to eat up to the anatomical capacity of their stomachs, but they replaced some of their cereals and vegetables with foods like fat and sugar, of high calorific value but of negligible bulk. The result was that, when the end of the first week of freedom came, two of the subjects were found to have been eating food providing them with about 1,500 calories a day more than their accustomed amount—and the result was an inevitable gain in weight."

Reducing-diet foods that are low in calories but quite high in content of water and indigestible cellulose, take care of the natural, unconscious desire for bulk quite adequately. Yet, there are many people who make complaints like these about reducing diets:

"I feel starved all the time." "They leave me weak and tired, no good for anything." "I'm so irritable when I diet that I'm not fit to live with." "I get all trembly and fatigued." "They take away all my strength, and I have no resistance left against colds and things."

Such opinions are sincere, and there is no doubt that some people actually *feel* the way they say. But are these complaints the result of mild starvation or grave physiological causes? The bulk of informed opinion says "no." As long as the reducer has excess fat, and his diet provides everything except calories, he can't starve or suffer physiological injury.

What are "hunger pangs"? They're supposed to be anguished yelps sent up by the stomach. But the stomach is quite unnecessary for true hunger sensations—can, in fact, be fooled by a couple of glasses of water. Dogs exhibit perfectly normal eating behavior although their stomachs have been totally removed. What is it, then, that acts like hunger and makes reducing a long unpleasantness for many? One specialist calls it "frustration of oral wishes," another, "memory of the pleasure of eating," and a third, "gustatory sensualism." Another considers it a bad sign if a patient plunges into an orgy of impassioned eating just before starting on a diet. This is taken to indicate deep rebellion against restriction and regimentation, and bodes ill for dietary persistence.

We can't pretend that there are easy, simple cures for resistances that have deep emotional roots. But we can make reasonable promises about the reducing diets you will meet on the next page, if your doctor has told you you must get rid of a few pounds:

They will not of themselves leave you weak and tired, irritable and cranky, run-down and fatigued, or truly hungry. They are indeed so packed with good nutrition that they can serve as a framework for better and more healthful eating for *everybody*, including people who want to gain weight. Not least important, they should be eaten with no sense of guilt or deprivation, enjoyed down to the last tasty morsel, to condition you to the very happy truth that permanent weight control does not mean that you must or should give up the pleasure of good eating.

Chapter 7

Better Homes & Gardens
meal plans

Now we come to the exciting moment when you are ready to begin your reducing diet. You are going to reduce by eating—controlled but satisfying eating. You probably have a good idea of how many pounds you want to lose, estimated from information given in the preceding chapter, and from advice your physician has given you. How *fast* can you lose fat? A fat loss of 1½ to 2 pounds a week is approved by most doctors as a safe and conservative reducing speed. (Weight loss may be greater, if water is lost from the tissues in addition to fat.)

The *Better Homes & Gardens* reducing diets that follow are designed to bring about fat losses up to about two pounds a week, a rate that your doctor will probably O.K. Reducing speed depends upon the *deficit* between the calories your food provides and the calories you burn up in bodily activities. For every deficit of 4,000 calories, you lose slightly more than one pound of fat. Obviously, the same reducing diet will not reduce everybody at precisely the same rate of speed, because of personal differences of energy expenditure and physical activity. The *Better Homes & Gardens* reducing diets come in three "speeds," of 1,000 calories, 1,250 calories, and 1,500 calories. The 1,000-calorie diets, of course, slim you faster than the 1,500-calorie ones. Yet the more ample 1,500-calorie diets are quite capable of slimming some people down at a desirable two-pounds-a-week rate, or even faster. Better talk it over with your doctor.

You can, if you wish, refer back to the previous chapter where we show you how you can figure your maintenance needs—the calories required to maintain normal weight. From these daily maintenance calories, *subtract* the calories of your reducing diet—1,000, 1,250, or 1,500 as the case may be. The result is your calorie *deficit*. Figure how many days of dieting it will take to build up a deficit of 4,000 calories. You should lose one pound of fat or a little more in that many days. Generally speaking, a 1,000-calorie diet will effect a fat loss of about two pounds a week in an average overweight woman who is moderately active.

How long can you stay on a diet?

You may notice that the *Better Homes & Gardens* reducing diets are not billed as Five Day, or Ten Day, or Fourteen Day diets. The reason is that you can, and should stay on them *as long as excess fat is present*. Not a day longer! When you have attained normal weight, you no longer have any useless surplus fat to make up for calories that reducing diets are deliberately designed *not* to provide. Then—happy days!—you need to get more calories from food, or else your body will have to steal them from vital organs, and that will make you very sick and very unhappy.

Another reason why no specific time limit is placed on the diets is that reducers who slim down on short-term diets are prone to feel that the battle of overweight is won, once and for all. It never is, or hardly ever. Fat will come right back again if eating is unrestrained and daily meals pile up a calorie surplus. *Permanent* weight control depends upon re-educating one's appetite and eating habits. Foods provided in the *Better Homes & Gardens* meal plans are those common to average American diets. That way the transition to higher calorie diets, after weight is reduced, will be easy and natural. Diets containing exotic "health foods" or strange and unusual things to eat are all too likely to make the reducer feel that there is some wonderful short-term magic in them. There is no such magic, and the road to lifetime weight control lies in intelligent eating of a wide variety of common and delicious foods of the familiar kinds provided by the following meals.

Incidentally, when you're eating the foods in these meal plans, enjoy every morsel of them. Don't believe for a minute that you ought to feel guilty because you aren't suffering, or because your taste buds are telling you, "This is delicious!"

How to use the diets

There's nothing fussy, tricky, or complicated about following our diet meals. Just go ahead and start eating. However, certain practical questions may occur to you as you put your reducing plan into action. Doubtless you already know the answers to many of these questions, but, for ready reference, we will discuss some of the things you may wonder about.

Cooking methods. Do not use methods that call for added fats or oils, such as frying, for calorie values are considerably increased. Broiling, boiling, poaching, baking, roasting, are suitable methods. Cut visible fat from meats if possible. Meat shrinks when cooked, losing some fat; collect fat drippings or skim off. To save vitamins and minerals in vegetables, cook in small amount of boiling water in a covered pan, or steam or pressure-cook them.

Try to include some *uncooked* fruits and vegetables every day—au naturel or in salads; citrus or other fruit juices. You can squeeze orange or grapefruit juice in advance, and store in a covered container in your refrigerator for two or three days, with almost no loss of vitamin C. *Frozen* fruits, juices, and vegetables retain vitamin and mineral values practically intact. Thaw according to directions on package. Store cans of frozen orange-juice concentrate in your freezer or freezing compartment of your refrigerator. *Canned* foods retain their nutrients so well, under modern processing methods, that it's personal choice, whether you use canned or fresh forms.

Table salt. Salt your food to your own taste, unless your doctor advises against it. Salt does not make fat, but in some people who are sick, it may hold abnormal amounts of water in the tissues.

Spices. There's no reason for any generally healthy person to shun spices. Maybe they've been maligned because they help to make even poor food palatable, and that goes against the grain of a puritanical conscience. Use them as liberally as you wish to add zest to your diet.

Flavor boosters that don't cost calories

Allspice	Lime	Pepper (white, black, red)
Almond extract	Mace	
Bay leaves	Mustard	Peppermint
Caraway	Mint	Pimiento
Curry	Monosodium	Poultry seasoning
Celery salt	glutamate	Sage
Chives	Mustard	Salt
Cinnamon	Noncaloric	Tabasco sauce
Dill	sweeteners	Thyme
Garlic	Nutmeg	Vanilla
Ginger	Onion salt	Vinegar
Herbs	Paprika	Worcestershire
Horse-radish	Parsley	sauce
Lemon		

Beverages. Drink as much water as you want; let thirst be your guide. You get some water from practically every food you eat, even from supposedly "dry" ones such as cereals. Water does not make fat, and water retention, which sometimes masks loss of fat, is not a matter of how much you drink but of physiological processes.

Black coffee and plain tea furnish no calories, can be taken according to taste. Use your milk quota in these beverages, if you wish, or a lemon slice with your tea.

Soda pop and the most popular kinds of soft drinks (except the no-calorie varieties) contain relatively large amounts of sugar that have to be added in a reducing diet. You may forget to count, but your body doesn't.

Sweeteners. Sodium and calcium cyclamates are medically accepted sweeteners of no caloric value that may be used freely as sugar substitutes in coffee and other foodstuffs. The cyclamates are especially suited for use in recipes that require heat in preparation. Saccharin is a much more concentrated sweetening agent. If a slightly bitter taste is noted, it probably means that too much saccharin was used; reduce the amount. These noncaloric sweeteners are available at drugstores without prescription. For the present, at least, some authorities believe that the use of these sweeteners should be restricted to those who need to reduce their intake of sweets.

Salad dressings. Salads play an important part in reducing diets, but the familiar delicious dressings that everybody likes run quite high in calories because of fat and oil content. You can use lemon juice, vinegar, salt and spices, without adding any calories worth counting,

and tomato juice is quite low in calories, too. Mir.
is not a food and contains no calories. But nutritionists
frown upon mineral oil as a dressing base because it tends
to interfere with assimilation of important oil-soluble
nutrients from foods. If you have to watch calories, a way
to solve the dressing problem is to make your own supply
from low-calorie recipes. Here are some good ones:

Rosy Dressing

1 cup water	½ teaspoon paprika
2 tablespoons enriched flour	½ teaspoon Worcestershire
½ cup vinegar	sauce
¼ cup catsup	⅛ teaspoon liquid sweetener
1 teaspoon horse-radish	1 clove garlic
1 teaspoon dry mustard	

Gradually stir water into flour. Cook over low heat, stirring constantly, until thick, about 5 minutes. Cool. Add
all other ingredients except garlic. Beat until smooth and
well blended. Add garlic. Cover, store in refrigerator.
Shake well before using. Makes 1⅔ cups. Total calories:
135. Per tablespoon: 5.

Calorie-counters Cooked Fruit Dressing

1 egg	¼ cup lemon juice, fresh,
1 egg yolk	frozen, or canned
½ cup pineapple juice	¼ teaspoon noncaloric liquid
	sweetener

Beat egg and egg yolk slightly. Add fruit juices and sweetener. Cook in double boiler over *hot, not boiling*, water,
stirring constantly, until thick. Cool. Makes ¾ cup. Total
calories: 215. Per tablespoon: 20.

Dieter's Cooked Dressing

2 teaspoons dry mustard	4 teaspoons cold water
1 teaspoon salt	¾ cup hot water
Dash paprika	1 tablespoon butter or
2 tablespoons sugar	margarine
½ tablespoon (½ envelope)	1 well-beaten egg
unflavored gelatin	¼ cup cider vinegar

Mix mustard, salt, paprika, and sugar. Soften gelatin in cold water. Add hot water to mustard mixture and stir until blended. Add softened gelatin and butter; stir till gelatin dissolves. Stir hot mixture slowly into beaten egg. Return to heat and cook, stirring constantly, until mixture begins to thicken. Remove from heat and stir in vinegar. Pour into jar and set aside to cool and thicken. Makes 1¼ cups. Total calories: 300. Per tablespoon: 15.

Now, there's nothing left but to start right in on your diet. Why wait until tomorrow? Some overweight people have been doing that for 20 years! If, as you read this, your next scheduled meal is dinner, start your diet with dinner. Or lunch, or breakfast. Change the order of foods that are listed for any one day, if you want to, but try to include at least a small portion of some complete protein, (milk, cheese, eggs, meat, fish, etc.) every time you eat. *Do* eat everything that is listed on the meal plans. One reason is that the foods are carefully selected to provide a balanced diet. Another reason, maybe more potent, is that you are going to have a pretty rough time convincing yourself that you "feel starved" on a diet, if you can't even eat all that is allowed.

If you pack a lunch box

It may seem to some reducers that it's an insuperable problem to pack a lunch box with foods of high nutritive quality, yet sufficiently low in calories to keep within dietary bounds. Not at all! That good old mainstay of the lunch box, the sandwich, is portable, palatable, and packable, and it can deliver a whale of a lot of protective nourishment at relatively low caloric cost. Low, at least, relative to the excellent protein, vitamins, and minerals provided.

The sandwich recipes below are pretty much equivalent to many of the main-course luncheon items served at restaurants. The difference is that in restaurants the meat, eggs, and vegetables look more impressive when isolated on plates in individual portions. All these sandwiches have good protein fillings, except the sliced-radish novelty (for lunch-box use, include a hard-cooked egg along with it).

You will note that low-calorie dressings are specified for use in the sandwich fillings. That's for reducers. Actually, these sandwiches are splendid good-nourishment items for improving the quality of packed lunches in general—the ones the youngsters carry to school, or Dad to the plant, or Sister to the office. For heartier eaters who have no reducing problem, make the sandwiches with mayonnaise, whipped, or other regular dressings, be more liberal with butter or margarine, add a bit of jelly or something sweet if it pleases the customer.

In addition to sandwiches, round out lunch-box quality, and increase stomach-satisfying quantity, by including milk, an orange, apple, pear, or other fruit in season, celery stalks, carrot strips, crisp slices of baby turnips.

Meat and fish sandwiches

1. Cooked ham, ground and mixed with pickle relish, chopped celery, chopped hard-cooked egg, dressing.*
2. Equal parts flaked tuna, crab meat, or lobster, and finely cut celery, moistened with dressing.
3. Liverwurst, chopped stuffed olives, dressing, with lettuce and rye bread.
4. Liverwurst, lettuce, and tomato on whole-wheat bread.
5. Chopped cooked chicken, finely cut celery, chopped sweet pickle, moistened with dressing.
6. Ground cooked meat, pickle relish or pickled onion, dressing, and prepared mustard or horse-radish.
7. Combine ½ cup finely chopped unpared cucumber, 1 teaspoon chopped chives, and one 7-ounce can shrimp, cleaned and minced. Add 1 tablespoon French dressing and 1 tablespoon salad dressing. Makes 1½ cups. Spread on bread cut crescent shape or use as a regular sandwich filling.

Cheese and egg sandwiches

1. Cottage cheese, minced green pepper, onion, salt, and paprika on whole-wheat bread.

*Editor's note: Use low-calorie dressings or use regular commercial dressings sparingly in all these sandwich fillings.

2. Eggs scrambled with minced onion and green pepper and a bit of finely chopped ham.

3. Chopped hard-cooked eggs, chopped dill pickle, and dressing, on leaf lettuce and rye bread.

4. Three chopped hard-cooked eggs, 2 tablespoons green onion, ¼ cup chopped green pepper, ½ cup chopped cucumber, and ½ teaspoon salt. Combine these ingredients with ¼ cup dressing.

Novelty sandwiches

1. Thinly sliced radishes on lightly buttered slices of whole-wheat bread.

2. To make Mock Pate de Foie Gras, put ½ pound cooked calves' liver through food chopper. Add 1 tablespoon lemon juice, 1 teaspoon Worcestershire sauce, 4 sprigs parsley, chopped, 1 teaspoon salt, 1 teaspoon chopped onion. Mix thoroughly with enough salad dressing to moisten. Makes 2 cups.

Sure, you can substitute

Someday, smack in the middle of your reducing diet, you may rummage in your refrigerator for some breast of chicken, specified for the day's dinner, and find nothing on hand but cold roast beef. Can you substitute the beef for the chicken?

Well, can you think of any reason why you shouldn't? Muscle meats are more or less equivalent to each other nutritionally. You are doubtless aware of that, and we're shamefaced about bringing up this matter of substitutions because it may seem ridiculously obvious to you. We wouldn't mention it, either, except that there are a few reducers who diet by dogma, follow menus slavishly, and are cast into dejection if they have to eat spinach on Tuesday when it's specified for Thursday.

You not only can substitute foods of similar quality for each other, but you should. Meat for fish, eggs for meat, potato for cereal, bread for rice, one green leafy vegetable or one root vegetable for another of the same type.

You will encounter discussions of comparative food values in various sections of this book, and it's quite easy to recognize general food classes so that diet substitutions can be made with confidence. During your first days or weeks of reducing, it is good to eat the menu-specified foods as faithfully as you can. But if some of yesterday's roast is left over, you can serve it for today's meat course without feeling that you have wrecked your program. And, as the weeks pass, experiment a little with substitutions. Then you'll be prepared to make intelligent diet decisions the rest of your life, and if you stick to your reducing program it's probably going to be a longer life so you might as well face it.

How to hold your losses

The day will come when you will have to stop reducing. That day arrives when your scales show your weight to be normal. It might be a dangerous day. You might kick over the traces, figuring you've won the decision, and go back to old eating habits that caused poundage in the first place. We don't think that this is too likely, if you have followed the *Better Homes & Gardens* reducing diets and discovered that good foods can be satisfying and delicious without being unduly fattening. But it's as well to be wary.

Stop and take stock. You are going to need enough calories to maintain your normal weight. Something must be added to the reducing diet that has served its purpose. What foods are you going to add to provide those calories?

You can take second helpings or larger servings of the foods you became accustomed to on your diet. Since they are selected for good balance, your added calories will come from good protective foods. Increase your quota of butter and margarine, bread, whole instead of skim milk, a little cream on breakfast cereals or in coffee. Add a modestly sweet dessert now and then, something you particularly like.

In short, increase your calorie intake gradually and with discretion, and more than ever, keep watching those scales! For it's much easier to *stay* at normal weight than to continually revert to strict diets to pare off pounds that have crept up unnoticed.

If the scales creep upward, three, four, or five pounds over normal weight, cut back a little on the food extras you have been adding. Skip a rich dessert, cut fatty foods down, but don't leave them out, apply the food knowledge you've gained by dieting, and you should be able to stay in shape for a lifetime.

Eat-all-you-want foods

If you are reducing, you can eat all you want of the following foods without increasing your calorie intake enough to make any practical difference—even if you gorge! They are 3-percent-carbohydrate vegetables, which give a very large amount of satisfying bulk but surprisingly few calories. There's no reason for getting up from the table with an empty, unsatisfied feeling if any one of these foods is served. An average half-cup serving supplies just about enough calories to take care of basal metabolic needs (when you're sleeping, resting, doing nothing) for only 15 mintues. This is true only if the vegetables are served without added sauces, creams, fats, oils, or sugars.

Asparagus	Cucumbers	Parsley
Young beans,	Endive	Radishes
green or wax	Escarole	Rhubarb
Broccoli	Greens: beet,	Romaine
Cabbage	dandelion,	Sauerkraut
Cauliflower	mustard, turnip	Spinach
Celery.	Kale	Summer squash
Chard	Lettuce	Tomatoes
Chicory	Mushrooms	Water cress

Weigh first thing in the morning

Reason: You're lighter then. You've been burning calories all night. *You may be losing fat* (in fact, will be if you're faithful to a sufficiently low-calorie diet) *although the scales don't show it.*

Water, which weighs more than fat, may be retained temporarily in the tissues. You may also lose water along with fat, so total weight loss is greater than actual fat loss. However, after a couple weeks—usually much sooner—water retention comes into balance, and the scales tell a true story of daily fat loss.

Don't eat when you are not hungry

This may sound silly, but we all eat at times when we're not hungry—television snacks, bridge-game sweets, nibbling just to break the day's routine. It doesn't take will power not to eat when we're not hungry.

Stop before you're full

This is one of the most important and least appreciated aids to sticking on a diet. Have you ever said, a few minutes after waddling away from a Thanksgiving dinner, "I ate too much!"? You didn't feel that way while eating. It takes a little while for food to be assimilated and give that full-up signal that we've had enough. If you keep on eating as long as things taste good going down, you're almost sure to overeat—what's worse, to eat more than you really want and certainly more than you're truly hungry for. On a reducing diet, of course, you can't overeat. But you may still think you're hungry immediately after finishing an allotted meal. Wait a few minutes before you hunt for something sweet to stave off "hunger pangs." As the meal begins to get into your blood where you can feel it (food in the stomach is not really *in* the body—just surrounded by it), you'll be pleasantly surprised to find that "hunger pangs" have gone and got lost.

Save a serving for a snack

If you just must eat something before you go to bed, or in the middle of an afternoon, let the snack be a serving from lunch or dinner (not breakfast) of the day's diet. You overdraw your diet, make repayment by not eating the "borrowed" food at regular mealtime.

Don't skip breakfast

If you do, you'll probably feel famished and have to steal a snack long before lunchtime. A reasonably good breakfast makes it much easier to stay on a diet.

You are absolutely certain to lose fat

If you are overweight, if your diet is sufficiently low in calories, if you don't cheat, nothing can stop you from losing excess fat.

Meal plans for
winter

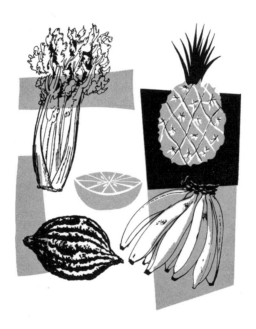

Wintertime is a fine time to start losing

weight! Your diet needn't be one of parsnips

and carrots daily. Because of modern freezing

and packaging wizardry, foods know no season

Winter $1,000$ *calories per day*

1st day | 2nd day

BREAKFAST

Chilled applesauce, ½ *cup*
Scrambled egg, 1
Enriched white toast, ½ *slice*
Butter, ½ *pat*
Skim milk, 1 *cup*

BREAKFAST

Unsweetened grapefruit
  juice, ½ *cup*
Whole bran, ¼ *cup*
Egg cooked in shell,
  your style, 1
Skim milk, 1 *cup*

LUNCH

Fat-free chicken broth, 1 *cup*
Roast veal, 3 *ounces*
Green beans, ½ *cup*
Perfection salad, ½ *cup*
Molasses cookies, 2
Skim milk, 1 *cup*

LUNCH

Cold pork loin, 1½ *ounces*
Broccoli, ½ *cup*
Salad of:
  Pineapple, 1 *slice*
  Cottage cheese,
    2 *tablespoons on* lettuce
Buttermilk, 1 *cup*

DINNER

Baked cod, 4 *ounces with*
  lemon wedge
Baked acorn squash, ½
Peas, ¾ *cup*
Fruit cup of:
  Orange sections, ½ *medium*
  Grapefruit, ¼ *medium*
Coffee

DINNER

Broiled beef patty, lean,
  3 *ounces*
Parsleyed potato, ½ *medium*
Butter, 1 *teaspoon*
Salad of:
  Sliced tomato, 1 *small*
  Cucumber, 6 *slices*
Dill pickle, 3 *slices*
Sliced orange, 1 *medium*
Coffee

Winter 1,000 *calories per day*

3rd day

BREAKFAST

Tangerine, 1 *medium*
Egg cooked in shell,
  your style, 1
Whole-wheat toast, 1 *slice*
Butter, ½ *pat*
Skim milk, 1 *cup*

LUNCH

Hot tomato juice, 1 *cup*
Casserole of:
  Diced chicken, 2 *ounces*
  Rice, ¼ *cup*
  Pimiento, ½ *medium*
  Green pepper, ½ *medium*
Spinach, *with* vinegar, ½ *cup*
Celery curls, 2 *stalks*
Pink grapefruit, ½ *medium*
Skim milk, 1 *cup*

DINNER

Baby beef liver, 3 *ounces*
Carrot coins, ½ *cup*
Cauliflower, ½ *cup*
Salad of:
  Tomato aspic, ⅓ *cup*
  Dieter's Cooked Dressing,
  1 *tablespoon on* lettuce
Pear, ½ *medium*
Tea

4th day

BREAKFAST

Chilled orange juice, ½ *cup*
Shredded wheat,
  1 *large biscuit*
Broiled Canadian bacon
  1 *slice*
Skim milk, 1 *cup*

LUNCH

Corned beef, *2 ounces*
Sauerkraut, ½ *cup*
Carrot curls, 1 *medium*
Baked custard, ½ *cup*
Skim milk, 1 *cup*

DINNER

Veal cutlet, 3 *ounces*
Mashed potato, ½ *cup*
Browned parsnips, ½ *cup*
Salad of:
  Club-style lettuce, 1″ *slice*
  Tomato slices, ½ *small*
  Rosy Dressing, 1 *tablespoon*
Baked apple, 1 *medium*
Coffee

Winter 1,250 *calories per day*

1 *st day*	2 *nd day*
BREAKFAST	**BREAKFAST**

Stewed apricots, ½ *cup*
Oatmeal, ½ *cup with*
  sugar, 1 *teaspoon*
Skim milk, 1 *cup*
	Unsweetened grapefruit
	  juice, ½ *cup*
	Canadian bacon, 2 *slices*
	Egg cooked in shell, 1
	Whole-wheat toast, 1 *slice*
	Coffee

LUNCH	**LUNCH**

Sandwich of:
  Grilled ground beef,
    lean, 3 *ounces*
  Whole-wheat toast, 1 *slice*
Sweet pickle, 1 *small*
Cauliflowerets, ½ *cup*
Carrot curls, ½ *medium*
Molasses cooky, 1
Skim milk, 1 *cup*
	Shrimp, 3 *ounces*
	Tossed green salad, 1 *cup*
	Salt bread sticks, 3
	Fruit cup of:
	  Banana, ⅓ *medium*
	  Orange slices, ½ *small*
	Skim milk, 1 *cup*

DINNER	**DINNER**

Baked pork chop, 3 *ounces*
Green beans, ½ *cup*
Salad of:
  Orange slices, 1 *small*
  Onion rings, 4
  Lettuce
Custard, ½ *cup*
Coffee
	Beef roast, 3 *ounces*
	Browned potato, 1 *medium*
	Broccoli, ½ *cup with*
	  lemon
	Sliced tomato, 1 *small*
	Raspberry sherbet, ½ *cup*
	Skim milk, 1 *cup*

Winter 1,250 *calories per day*

3rd day | 4th day

BREAKFAST

Tomato juice, ½ *cup*
Broiled Canadian bacon,
  2 *slices*
Scrambled egg, 1
Coffee

BREAKFAST

Broiled grapefruit, ½ *medium*
Toast, 1 *slice*
Butter, ½ *pat*
Puffed cereal, 1 *cup*
Skim milk, 1 *cup*

LUNCH

Veal patty, 3 *ounces*
Peas, ½ *cup*
Julienne carrots, 1 *medium*
Cabbage, *shredded,* ½ *cup*
  Dieter's Cooked Dressing,
  1 *tablespoon*
Sliced orange, 1 *small*
Skim milk, 1 *cup*

LUNCH

Browned spiced ham, 2 *ounces*
Asparagus spears, 6
Sliced hard-cooked egg, 1
Pear, ½
Skim milk, 1 *cup*

DINNER

Roast turkey, 4 *ounces*
Baked acorn squash,
  ½ *medium*
Beet slices ½ *cup*
Baked apple, 1 *medium*
Skim milk, 1 *cup*

DINNER

Broiled club steak, 3 *ounces*
Carrots, ½ *cup*
Green beans, *seasoned with*
  garlic, ½ *cup*
Salad of:
  Cottage cheese, ¼ *cup on*
  lettuce
Prune whip, ½ *cup*
Coffee

Winter 1,500 *calories per day*

1st day	2nd day
BREAKFAST	**BREAKFAST**
Stewed prunes, unsweetened, 8 *medium* Shirred egg, 1 Crisp bacon, 2 *slices* Buttered muffin, 1 Skim milk, 1 *cup*	Orange juice, ½ *cup* Rice flakes, 1 *cup* Banana, ½ *medium* Egg cooked in shell, 1 Buttered bread, 1 *slice* Skim milk, 1 *cup*
LUNCH	**LUNCH**
Sandwich of: 　Whole-wheat bread, 2 *slices* 　American cheese, 1 *ounce* 　Sliced tomato, 1 *medium* Tossed green salad, 1 *cup* 　Rosy Dressing, 1 *tablespoon* Lemon sherbet, ⅓ *cup* Skim milk, 1 *cup*	Stewed chicken, 2 *ounces* Noodles, ½ *cup* Asparagus, ½ *cup* Perfection salad, ½ *cup* Apple, 1 *medium* Skim milk, 1 *cup*
DINNER	**DINNER**
Roast veal, 3 *ounces* Whole kernel corn, ½ *cup* Cauliflower, ⅓ *cup* Salad of: 　Grapefruit *and* orange 　sections, ½ *medium* 　*each on* lettuce Strawberry gelatin, ½ *cup* Coffee	Broiled ham steak, 3 *ounces* Stuffed baked potato, 　½ *medium* Brussels sprouts, ½ *cup* Carrot curls, ½ *medium* Celery sticks, 3 *stalks* Gingerbread, 2″ *cube* Coffee

Winter $1{,}500$ *calories per day*

3rd day | ## 4th day

BREAKFAST	**BREAKFAST**
Tangerine, 1 *medium*	Grapefruit sections, 1 *cup*
Vienna sausage, 2 *ounces*	Oatmeal, ½ *cup with*
Scrambled egg, 1	sugar, ½ *teaspoon*
Whole-wheat toast, 1 *slice*	raisins, 1 *tablespoon*
Skim milk, 1 *cup*	Canadian bacon, 2 *ounces*
	Skim milk, 1 *cup*
LUNCH	**LUNCH**
Baked salmon steak, 4 *ounces*	Boiled dinner of:
with lemon wedge	Corned beef, 2 *ounces*
Green beans, ½ *cup*	Cabbage, ½ *cup*
Chef's salad bowl, 1 *cup*	Carrot, 1 *medium*
Rosy Dressing, 1 *tablespoon*	Salad of ½ *cup*
Carrot strips, ½ *medium*	cherry gelatin *with*
Plums, 2	celery *and* apple
Skim milk, 1 *cup*	Rye bread, 1 *slice*
	Butter, ½ *pat*
	Baked custard, ½ *cup*
DINNER	**DINNER**
Meat loaf, 1 *slice*	Lamb chop, *3 ounces*
Baked potato, 1 *medium*	Minted peas, ½ *cup*
Beets, ½ *cup*	Tomato aspic salad, ⅓ *cup*
Orange salad, 1 *medium on*	Pear, 1 *medium*
endive	Skim milk, 1 *cup*
Crescent roll, 1	Tea
Butter, ½ *pat*	
Maple chiffon cake, 2″ *wedge*	
Coffee	

Meal plans for
spring

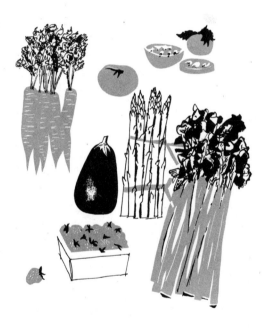

Spring is a wonderful season for dieters! Take

advantage of this season's plentiful offerings of

straight-from-the-garden vegetables, and you'll

forget your notions about meager reducing meals

Spring 1,000 *calories per day*

# 1 *st day*	# 2 *nd day*
BREAKFAST	**BREAKFAST**
Grapefruit juice, ½ *cup* Broiled ham, 2 *ounces* Toast, 1 *slice* Butter, ½ *pat* Skim milk, 1 *cup*	Black raspberries, ½ *cup* Puffed cereal, 1 *cup* Broiled Canadian bacon, 1 *slice* Skim milk, 1 *cup*
LUNCH	**LUNCH**

Salad of:
  Shrimp, 5
  Lettuce, 2 *leaves*
  Celery, 3 *small stalks*
  Radishes, 4 *small*
  Green onion, 1
  Hard-cooked egg, 1
  Rosy Dressing, 2 *tablespoons*
Saltines, 2 *squares*
Low-calorie limeade, 1 *cup*
	Fat-free chicken broth,
	  1 *cup*
	Cold, sliced tongue, 2 *ounces*
	Salad of:
	  Cottage cheese, ¼ *cup*
	  with sliced orange,
	  ½ *medium on* lettuce
	Buttermilk, 1 *cup*

DINNER	**DINNER**

Roast beef, 3 *ounces*
Sliced beets, ½ *cup*
Chef's salad, 1 *cup with*
  lemon
Carrot curls, ½ *medium*
Fresh pineapple, ½ *cup*
Skim milk, 1 *cup*
	Broiled sirloin steak, 4 *ounces*
	Garden green beans, ½ *cup*
	Butter, ½ *pat*
	Green salad, ½ *cup*
	  with Rosy Dressing,
	  1 *tablespoon*
	Custard, ½ *cup*
	Coffee

Spring 1,000 *calories per day*

3rd day

BREAKFAST

Tomato juice, ½ *cup*
Egg cooked in shell,
your style, 1
Toast, ½ *slice*
Skim milk, 1 *cup*

LUNCH

Broiled beef patty, lean,
3 *ounces*
Relish plate of:
Dill-pickle slices, 6
Celery hearts, 2
Radish roses, 4
Green onions, 2
Carrot curls, ½ *medium*
Strawberries, ½ *cup*
Skim milk, 1 *cup*

DINNER

Roast veal, 3 *ounces*
Peas, ½ *cup*
Salad of:
Orange, ½ *medium and*
grapefruit sections ¼
medium on lettuce
Muffin, 1
Butter, ½ *pat*
Coffee

4th day

BREAKFAST

Fresh strawberries, ½ *cup*
Puffed cereal, 1 *cup*
Poached egg, 1
Skim milk, 1 *cup*

LUNCH

Consomme, 1 *cup*
Sandwich of:
Liverwurst, 2 *ounces*
Rye bread, 1 *slice*
Butter, ½ *pat*
Asparagus, ½ *cup*
Rhubarb sauce, ½ *cup*
noncaloric sweetener
Buttermilk, 1 *cup*

DINNER

Roast lamb, 3 *ounces*
Green beans *seasoned with*
garlic, ½ *cup*
Club-style lettuce, 1″ *slice*
and green-pepper rings
Dieter's Cooked Dressing,
1 *tablespoon*
Sliced oranges, 1½ *medium*
Tea

122

Spring 1,250 *calories per day*

1st day

BREAKFAST

Blueberries, ½ *cup*
Corn flakes, 1 *cup*
Poached egg, 1
Skim milk, 1 *cup*

LUNCH

Cold, sliced chicken, 2 *ounces*
  on lettuce
Green beans, ½ *cup*
Tomato aspic salad, ⅓ *cup*
Radishes, 4 *small*
Popover, 1
Butter, ½ *pat*
Sliced orange, 1 *medium*
Skim milk, 1 *cup*

DINNER

Lamb chop, 3 *ounces*
Compote of vegetables:
  Carrot, 1
  Peas, ⅓ *cup*
  Cabbage, ⅔ *cup*
Salad of:
  Pineapple, 1 *slice*
  Cottage cheese, ¼ *cup*
Peanut-butter cooky, 1
Coffee

2nd day

BREAKFAST

Orange juice ½ *cup*
Broiled ham slice, 2 *ounces*
Bran muffin, 1
Butter, 1 *pat*
Skim milk, 1 *cup*

LUNCH

Jellied consomme, 1 *cup*
Tuna 3 *ounces on*
  lettuce
Sliced tomato, 1 *small*
Rhubarb sauce, ½ *cup*
  noncaloric sweetener
Skim milk, 1 *cup*

DINNER

Roast beef, 3 *ounces*
Mashed potatoes, ½ *cup*
Broccoli, ½ *cup*
Lettuce, 1″ *slice with*
  lemon
Strawberries, 1 *cup*
Coffee

Spring 1,250 *calories per day*

3rd day

BREAKFAST

Stewed prunes, unsweet-
    ened, 4 *medium*
Farina, ½ *cup*
Sugar, ½ *teaspoon*
Egg cooked in shell, 1
Skim milk, 1 *cup*

LUNCH

Frankfurter, 1, *split,*
    filled with ¼ *cup* mashed
    potatoes *and broiled*
Dill-pickle *slices*, 3
Celery curls, 3 *stalks*
Carrot sticks, ½ *medium*
Red raspberries, ½ *cup*
Skim milk, 1 *cup*

DINNER

Broiled chicken, ½ *broiler*
Steamed rice, ½ *cup*
Asparagus spears, 6
Salad of:
    Orange, 1 *medium, on* endive
    Sponge cake, 2″ *cube*
Coffee

4th day

BREAKFAST

Grapefruit, *medium,* ½
Scrambled egg, 1
Canadian bacon, 2 *slices*
Popover, 1
Butter, 1 *pat*
Skim milk, 1 *cup*

LUNCH

Hot tomato juice, 1 *cup*
Grilled sandwich of:
    Enriched white bread,
        2 *slices*
    American cheese, 1 *ounce*
Green beans, ½ *cup*
Fruit cup of:
    Strawberries, ½ *cup*
    Pineapple, ½ *cup*
Skim milk, 1 *cup*

DINNER

Baked perch fillet, 3 *ounces*
    with lemon wedge, paprika
Stuffed baked potato,
    ½ *medium*
Cabbage-pepper slaw, ½ *cup*
    Dieter's Cooked Dressing,
        1 *tablespoon*
Baked custard, ½ *cup*
Coffee

Spring 1,500 *calories per day*

1 *st day*	2 *nd day*
BREAKFAST	**BREAKFAST**
Pineapple juice, ½ *cup* Egg cooked in the shell, 1 Crisp bacon, 1 *slice* Raisin toast, 1 *slice* Butter, 1 *pat* Skim milk, 1 *cup*	Sliced orange, 1 *medium* Shredded wheat, 1 *large biscuit* Vienna sausage, 2 *ounces* Skim milk, 1 *cup*
LUNCH	**LUNCH**

Chicken broth, 1 *cup*
Omelet *with* mushrooms,
   1 *serving*
Sliced tomato, 1 *small*
Chef's salad, 1 *cup*
Roll, 1 *small*
Butter, ½ *pat*
Strawberry-rhubarb com-
   pote, ½ *cup, noncaloric sweetener*
Skim milk, 1 *cup*
	Cold roast beef, 3 *ounces*
	Salad of:
	   Lettuce, ¼ *head*
	   Rosy Dressing, 1 *tablespoon*
	   Hard-cooked egg, *sliced*, 1
	   Cottage cheese, ¼ *cup*
	   Tomato, 1 *medium*,
	Buttered bread, ½ *slice*
	Oatmeal cooky, 1
	Skim milk, 1 *cup*

DINNER	**DINNER**

Veal cutlet, 3 *ounces*
Parsleyed potato, 1 *medium*
Butter, ½ *pat*
Asparagus, 6 *spears*
Orange *and* grapefruit *sections*,
   ½ *medium, each, on* lettuce
Sponge cake, 2″ *cube*
Coffee
	Roast lamb, 3 *ounces*
	Spiced apricot, 1
	Mashed potatoes, ½ *cup*
	Butter, 1 *pat*
	Green beans, ½ *cup*
	Salad of:
	   Celery *and* apple *in*
	      cherry gelatin, ½ *cup*
	Fresh pineapple, ½ *cup*
	Coffee

Spring 1,500 *calories per day*

3rd day

BREAKFAST

Pink grapefruit, ½
Egg cooked in shell,
 your style, 1
Toast, 1 *slice*
Butter, ½ *pat*
Skim milk, 1 *cup*

LUNCH

Beef-vegetable soup, 1 *cup*
Salad of:
 Lettuce, 2 *large leaves*
 Hard-cooked egg, 1 *sliced*
 Onion, 1 *slice in rings*
 Rosy Dressing, 1 *tablespoon*
Hard roll, 1
Butter, ½ *pat*
Royal Ann cherries, ½ *cup*
Skim milk, 1 *cup*

DINNER

Baked ham, 3 *ounces*
Spiced peach, ½
Oven-browned potato,
 1 *medium*
Small peas, ¼ *cup*
Carrots, ½ *cup*
Fresh spinach, ½ *cup with*
 vinegar
Lemon chiffon cake, 2″ *wedge*
Coffee

4th day

BREAKFAST

Black raspberries, ½ *cup*
Bran flakes, ½ *cup*
Crisp bacon, 2 *slices*
Toast, 1 *slice*
Butter, ½ *pat*
Skim milk, 1 *cup*

LUNCH

Sandwich of:
 Broiled beef patty, lean,
  3 *ounces*
 American cheese, 1 *ounce*
 Toasted bun, 1
Dill pickle, 2 *slices*
Fruit gelatin, ⅓ *cup*
Skim milk, 1 *cup*

DINNER

Broiled chicken, ¼ *broiler*
Parsleyed potato, 1 *medium*
Carrot coins, ½ *cup*
Strawberry shortcake of:
 Biscuit, 1
 Berries, ½ *cup*
Coffee

Meal plans for
summer

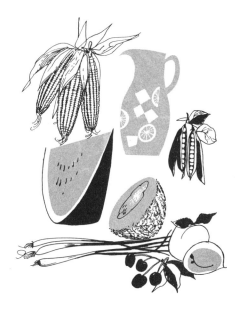

Summer couldn't be better for you, the reducer!

Treat yourself to all the wonderful melons and

berries—a fine source of vitamins and minerals.

Eat your fill and plan meals around them

Summer $1,000$ *calories per day*

1 *st day*	**2** *nd day*
BREAKFAST	**BREAKFAST**
Pineapple chunks, ½ *cup* Egg cooked in shell, *your style,* 1 Bran muffin, 1 Butter, 1 *teaspoon* Skim milk, 1 *cup*	Fresh apricots, 3 *medium* Scrambled egg, 1 *with* mushrooms, 2 *tablespoons* Whole-wheat toast, ½ *slice* Skim milk, 1 *cup*
LUNCH	**LUNCH**
Tomato juice, ½ *cup* Shrimp, 3 *ounces* Lemon wedge Celery, 3 *stalks* Carrot sticks, ¼ *cup* Pear, ½ *medium* Iced tea	Liverwurst, 2 *ounces* Boiled ham, 1 *ounce* Carrot coins, 1 *medium* Bread, 1 *slice* Butter, 1 *teaspoon* Red raspberries, ½ *cup* Skim milk, 1 *cup*
DINNER	**DINNER**
Jellied consomme, 1 *cup* Roast beef, 2 *ounces* Summer squash, ½ *cup* Peas, ¾ *cup* Melon-ball cup, ½ *cup* Honeydew, watermelon, cantaloupe Skim milk, 1 *cup*	Roast chicken, 3 *ounces* Green beans, ½ *cup* Shredded cabbage, ½ *cup* Dieter's Cooked Dressing, 1 *tablespoon* Sliced tomato, 1 *medium* Watermelon wedge, ¾″x10″ Iced tea

128

Summer 1,000 *calories per day*

3rd day

BREAKFAST

Rhubarb, ½ *cup*
  noncaloric sweetener,
Egg cooked in shell, 1
Bran muffin, 1
Butter, ½ *pat*
Skim milk, 1 *cup*

LUNCH

Broiled chicken livers,
  3 *ounces*
Coleslaw, ½ *cup*
Carrot sticks, ½ *medium*
Deviled egg, 1, *with* vinegar
  and low calorie dressing
Radish roses, 2
Melba toast, 1 *slice*
Blueberries, ½ *cup*
Low-calorie lemonade, 1 *cup*

DINNER

Veal cutlet, 3 *ounces*
Parsleyed potato, ½ *medium*
Tomato aspic, ⅓ *cup*
Sliced peach, 1 *medium*
Skim milk, 1 *cup*

4th day

BREAKFAST

Cantaloupe, ½ 5″ melon
Broiled Canadian bacon,
  2 *slices*
Graham crackers, 2
Skim milk, 1 *cup*

LUNCH

Liver, 2 *ounces*
Melba toast, ½ *slice*
Pear, ½
Camembert cheese, 1 *ounce*
Skim milk, 1 *cup*

DINNER

Steak, 3 *ounces*
Green beans, *seasoned with*
  garlic, ½ *cup*
Pineapple, ½ *cup*
Skim milk, 1 *cup*

Summer $1,250$ *calories per day*

1 *st day*

BREAKFAST

Black raspberries, ½ *cup*
Whole bran, ½ *cup*
Poached egg, 1
Skim milk, 1 *cup*

LUNCH

Frankfurters, 2
Green beans, *seasoned with*
  garlic, ½ *cup*
Bread, 1 *slice*
Butter, ½ *pat*
Peach, 1 *medium*
Skim milk, 1 *cup*

DINNER

Sirloin steak, 3 *ounces*
Spinach, ½ *cup with* vinegar
Chive cottage cheese, ½ *cup*
  on lettuce
Whole-wheat bread, 1 *slice*
Butter, ½ *pat*
Cantaloupe, ½ *medium*
Iced tea

2 *nd day*

BREAKFAST

Prunes, 4 *medium*
Crisp bacon, 2 *slices*
French toast, 1 *slice*
Jelly, 2 *teaspoons*
Skim milk, 1 *cup*

LUNCH

Sandwich of:
  Peanut butter, 2 *tablespoons*
  Lettuce, 2 *leaves*
  Sweet pickles, 2 *small*
  Enriched white bread,
    2 *slices*
Celery, 3 *stalks*
Bing cherries, ½ *cup*
Skim milk, 1 *cup*

DINNER

Broiled baby-beef liver,
  3 *ounces*
Perfection salad, ½ *cup in*
  pepper rings, ½ *medium*
Diced carrots, ½ *cup*
Butter, ½ *pat*
Apricots, 3
Iced coffee

Summer 1,250 *calories per day*

3rd day | 4th day

BREAKFAST

Blueberries, ½ *cup*
Corn flakes, 1 *cup*
Crisp Canadian bacon,
  2 *slices*
Skim milk, 1 *cup*

LUNCH

Chicken salad, ½ *cup*
Hard-cooked egg, 1
Sliced tomato, 1 *medium*
Crisp rye wafers, 2
Strawberry-rhubarb com-
  pote, ½ *cup*
  noncaloric sweetener
Skim milk, 1 *cup*

DINNER

Veal steak, 3 *ounces*
Mashed potatoes, ½ *cup*
Peas, ½ *cup* and carrots,
  1 *medium*
Coleslaw, 1 *cup*
Dieter's Cooked Dressing,
  1 *tablespoon*
Graham cracker, 1 *small*
Watermelon slice, ¾"x10"
Iced coffee

BREAKFAST

Tomato juice, ¾ *cup*
Scrambled egg, 1
Toast, 1 *slice*
Butter, ½ *pat*
Skim milk, 1 *cup*

LUNCH

Open-face sandwich of:
  Bread, 1 *slice*
  Swiss cheese, 2 *slices*
  Tomato slice, 1 *medium*
Lettuce, 1" *slice*
  Dieter's Cooked Dressing,
  1 *tablespoon*
Sliced peach, 1 *medium*
Skim milk, 1 *cup*

DINNER

Lobster, 3 *ounces*
Green lima beans, ½ *cup*
Caesar salad, *garnished with*
  1 hard-cooked egg
Strawberry shortcake of:
  Biscuit, 1
  Strawberries, ½ *cup*
Iced tea

Summer 1,500 *calories per day*

1 *st day* | 2 *nd day*

BREAKFAST

Honeydew, 2″ *wedge*
Crisp bacon, 2 *slices*
Poached egg, 1
Raisin toast, 1 *slice*
Butter, 1 *pat*
Skim milk 1 *cup*

BREAKFAST

Grapefruit juice, ½ *cup*
Scrambled egg, 1
  mushrooms, 2 *tablespoons*
Blueberry muffin, 1
Butter, ½ *pat*
Skim milk, 1 *cup*

LUNCH

Club sandwich of:
  Bread, 3 *thin slices*
  Butter, 1 *pat*
  Lettuce, 2 *leaves*
  Tomato, 1 *small*
  Chicken, 2 *ounces*
  Boiled ham, 1 *ounce*
Carrot curls, ½ *medium* carrot
Cauliflowerets, ¼ *cup*
Skim milk, 1 *cup*

LUNCH

Tuna salad, ½ *cup*
Sliced tomato, 1 *small*
Roll, 1
Butter, ½ *pat*
Sponge cake, 2″ *cube*
Skim milk, 1 *cup*

DINNER

Shrimp, 3 *ounces*
French fries, 8 *pieces*
Green beans, ½ *cup*
Chef's salad, 1 *cup*
Rosy Dressing, 1 *tablespoon*
Sundae of:
  Peach, ½ *sliced*
  Ice cream, ½ *cup*
Iced tea

DINNER

Broiled beef patty, lean,
  3 *ounces*
Peas, ½ *cup*
Corn on the cob, 1 *medium ear*
Lettuce, 1″ *medium slice*
  low-calorie dressing,
  1 *tablespoon*
Butter, 1 *pat*
Orange sherbet, ½ *cup*
Low-calorie lemonade, 1 *cup*

132

Summer $1,500$ *calories per day*

3rd day

BREAKFAST

Pineapple, 1½ *slices*
Ham slice, 1 *ounce*
Corn muffin, 1
Butter, ½ *pat*
Skim milk, 1 *cup*

LUNCH

Fruit plate of:
  ½ orange *and* ½ grape-
    fruit *in sections*
  Cottage cheese, ½ *cup*
  Chilled grapes, 1 *cup*
Brown bread, 1 *slice*
Butter, ½ *pat*
Skim milk, 1 *cup*

DINNER

Lamb chop, 3 *ounces*
Parsleyed potato, 1 *medium*
Broccoli, ½ *cup*
Cucumbers *and* onions,
  6 *slices of each in* vinegar
Apricots, 3
Iced tea

4th day

BREAKFAST

Orange juice, ½ *cup*
Poached egg, 1
Toast, 1 *slice*
Jam, 1 *tablespoon*
Skim milk, 1 *cup*

LUNCH

Jellied consomme, 1 *cup*
Salmon souffle, ¾ *cup*
Caesar salad, 1 *cup with*
  lemon juice
Rye bread, 1 *slice*
Butter, 1 *pat*
Plum, 1
Skim milk, 1 *cup*

DINNER

Picnic of:
  Chicken leg, 1
  Potato salad, ½ *cup*
    in tomato cup, 1 *small*
  Bread, 1 *slice*
  Butter, 1 *pat*
  Watermelon wedge, 4"x8"
  Iced coffee

Meal plans for
fall

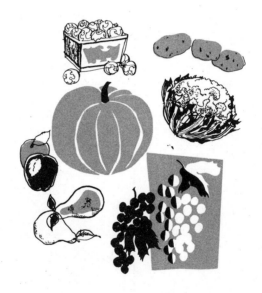

If fall is now, now is the time to start losing weight. Tomorrow, next week, or next month won't be better. Each season offers an exciting variety of foods; dieting will never be dull

Fall   1,000 *calories per day*

1st day

BREAKFAST

Orange, 1 *small*
Egg cooked in shell,
  your style, 1
Toast, 1 *slice*
Butter, ½ *pat*
Skim milk, 1 *cup*

LUNCH

Fat-free chicken broth, 1 *cup*
Jellied beef tongue, 4 *ounces*
Seven-minute cabbage,
  ½ *cup*
Diced carrot, 1 *medium*
Sliced tomato, 1 *small*
Cantaloupe, ½ *medium*
Skim milk, 1 *cup*

DINNER

Round steak, 3 *ounces*
Green lima beans, ¼ *cup*
Broccoli, ½ *cup*
Pineapple tidbits, ½ *cup*
Coffee

2nd day

BREAKFAST

Stewed prunes, *unsweetened*,
  4 medium
Farina, ½ *cup*
Sugar, ½ *teaspoon*
Canadian bacon, 1 *slice*
Skim milk, 1 *cup*

LUNCH

Hot tomato juice, *1 cup*
Broiled baby-beef liver,
  2 ounces
Green beans, ½ *cup*
Salad of:
  ½ medium orange *and* ¼
    grapefruit, *in sections*
    on lettuce
Buttermilk, 1 *cup*

DINNER

Roast chicken, 4 *ounces*
Mashed squash, ½ *cup*
Cauliflower, ½ *cup*
Carrot curls, ½ *medium*
Celery sticks, 2 *small stalks*
Baked custard, ½ *cup*
Skim milk, 1 *cup*

Fall 1,000 *calories per day*

3rd day

BREAKFAST

Stewed dried peaches,
  unsweetened, ⅓ *cup*
Poached egg, 1
  on toast, 1 *slice*
Butter, 1 *teaspoon*
Skim milk, 1 *cup*

LUNCH

Broiled Canadian bacon,
  2 *slices*
Sauerkraut, ½ *cup*
Salad of:
  Pear half
  Grated cheese, 1 *tablespoon*
  on lettuce
Skim milk, 1 *cup*

DINNER

Roast veal, 3 *ounces*
Carrot, 1 *medium*
Whole kernel corn, ¼ *cup*
Tomato, 1 *small*
Melba toast, ½ *slice*
Grapefruit, ½ *medium*
Coffee

4th day

BREAKFAST

Orange juice, ½ *cup*
Raisin bran flakes, ½ *cup*
Scrambled egg, 1
Skim milk, 1 *cup*

LUNCH

Consomme, 1 *cup*
Saltines, 2 *squares*
Cold sliced turkey, 2 *ounces*
Relish plate of:
  Cauliflowerets, ¼ *cup*
  Celery sticks, 3 *stalks*
  Tomato wedge, ¼ *medium*
Pink grapefruit, ½ *medium*
Skim milk, 1 *cup*

DINNER

Broiled beef patty, lean,
  3 *ounces*
Peas, ½ *cup*
Salad of:
  Grated carrot, ¼ *cup*
  Lettuce, 1″ *slice with* Rosy
    Dressing, 1 *tablespoon*
Sliced peach, 1 *medium*
Iced Tea

Fall   1,250 *calories per day*

1 *st day*

BREAKFAST

Grapefruit, ½ *medium*
Poached egg, 1
Whole-wheat toast, 1 *slice*
Butter, ½ *pat*
Skim milk, 1 *cup*

LUNCH

Sandwich of:
  Ham, 2 *ounces*
  Swiss cheese, ½ *slice*
  Lettuce, 1 *leaf*
  Rye bread, 1 *slice*
Dill pickles, 3 *slices*
Stewed apricots, ¼ *cup*
Skim milk, 1 *cup*

DINNER

Meat loaf, 1 *slice*
Baked potato, 1 *medium*
Diced carrots, ½ *cup*
Salad of:
  Sliced tomato, ½ *small*
  Cucumber, 6 *slices*
Angel cake, 2″ *wedge*
Coffee

2 *nd day*

BREAKFAST

Sliced orange, 1 *medium*
Canadian bacon, 2 *slices*
Bran muffin, 1
Butter, ½ *pat*
Jelly, 1 *teaspoon*
Skim milk, 1 *cup*

LUNCH

Salmon souffle, ¾ *cup*
Club-style lettuce, 1″ *slice*
  Pepper rings
  Lemon wedge
Tokay grapes, ¼ *cup*
Skim milk, 1 *cup*

DINNER

Roast veal, 3 *ounces*
Acorn squash, ½ *medium*
Butter, 1 *pat*
Green beans, ½ *cup*
Ambrosia salad, ⅓ *cup of:*
  bananas, oranges, dates,
  lemon juice, and coconut
Blue cheese, 1-*ounce wedge with*
  saltines, 2 *squares*
Coffee

Fall

1,250 *calories per day*

3rd day

BREAKFAST

Pineapple juice, ½ *cup*
Oatmeal, ½ *cup*
Sugar, ½ *teaspoon*
Skim milk, 1 *cup*

LUNCH

Tomato juice, 1 *cup*
Saltines, 2 *squares*
Cold plate of:
  Sardines, 2 *ounces*
  Deviled egg, 1 *with*
    Dieter's Cooked
    Dressing
  Radishes, 4 *small*
Apple, 1 *medium*
Skim milk, 1 *cup*

DINNER

Lamb chop, 3 *ounces*
Mashed potato, ⅓ *cup*
Minted peas, ½ *cup and*
  carrots, ¼ *cup*
Red cabbage, ½ *cup with*
  Dieter's Cooked
  Dressing, 1 *tablespoon*
Grapefruit, ½ *medium*
Coffee

4th day

BREAKFAST

Warm baked apple, 1 *small*
Scrambled egg, 1
Toast, ½ *slice*
Butter, ½ *pat*
Skim milk, 1 *cup*

LUNCH

Pork liver, 3 *ounces*
Onions, ½ *cup*
Saltines, 2 *squares*
Fruit cup of:
  Grapefruit *and* orange
  sections, ¼ *cup each in*
  ginger ale, 1 *tablespoon*
Skim milk, 1 *cup*

DINNER

Baked ham, 3 *ounces*
Parsleyed potato, 1 *medium*
Butter, 1 *pat*
Spinach, ½ *cup*
Pumpkin custard ½ *cup*
  (*pie filling, no crust*)
Coffee

138

Fall

1,500 *calories per day*

1st day

BREAKFAST

Tomato juice, ½ *cup*
Shredded wheat,
  1 *large biscuit*
Bran muffin, 1
Butter, 1 *pat*
Skim milk, 1 *cup*

LUNCH

Vegetable soup, 1 *cup*
Sandwich of:
  Egg, 1 *hard-cooked*
  Dieter's Cooked Dressing,
    1 *tablespoon*
  Rye bread, 2 *slices*
  Lettuce, 1 *leaf*
Carrot, 1 *cut in strips*
Orange, 1 *small*
Skim milk, 1 *cup*

DINNER

Roast beef, 3 *ounces*
Franconia potato, 1 *medium*
Brussels sprouts, ½ *cup*
Caesar salad, 1 *cup*
Saltines, 2 *squares*
Camembert cheese, 1 *ounce*
Coffee

2nd day

BREAKFAST

Orange juice, ½ *cup*
Crisp bacon, 2 *strips*
Scrambled egg, 1 *with*
  mushrooms, 2 *tablespoons*
Buttered toast, 1 *slice*
Coffee

LUNCH

Broiled baby-beef liver,
  3 *ounces*
Broiled tomato halves,
  2 *small*
Lettuce, 1" *slice*
  Rosy Dressing, 1 *tablespoon*
Banana, 1 *medium*
Skim milk, 1 *cup*

DINNER

Roast chicken, 4 *ounces*
Baked potato, 1 *medium*
Peas and carrots, ¼ *cup each*
Perfection salad, ½ *cup*
Roll, 1
Butter, 1 *pat*
Plums, 2
Green grapes, ¼ *cup*
Skim milk, 1 *cup*

Fall

1,500 *calories per day*

3rd day

BREAKFAST

Grapefruit, ½ *medium*
Broiled Canadian bacon,
  2 *slices*
Toast, 1 *slice*
Butter, 1 *pat*
Skim milk, 1 *cup*

LUNCH

Sandwich of:
  Broiled beef patty, lean,
    3 *ounces*
  Toasted bun, ½
Chef's salad, 1 *cup*, with
  lemon juice
Apple, 1 *medium*
Skim milk, 1 *cup*

DINNER

Veal chops, 3 *ounces*
Sweet potato, ½ *cup*
Green beans, ½ *cup*
Sliced tomato, 1 *small*
Baked custard, ½ *cup*
Coffee

4th day

BREAKFAST

Orange, 1 *medium sliced*
Crisp bacon, 2 *slices*
Poached egg, 1
Whole-wheat toast, 1 *slice*
Butter, ½ *pat*
Coffee

LUNCH

Oyster stew, ¾ *cup with*
  3 oysters
Oyster crackers, 10
Celery heart, 3 *stalks*
Cheddar cheese, 1″ *cube*
Olives, 3
Sliced tomato, 1 *medium*
Canned cherries, ½ *cup*
Coffee

DINNER

Meat-stuffed green pepper
Creamed potatoes, ⅓ *cup*
Julienne carrots, 2 *medium*
Salad of:
  Apple wedges, ¼ *medium*
  Grapefruit *sections*,
    ¼ *small on* lettuce
Sponge cake, 2″ *cube*
Skim milk, 1 *cup*

How to count calories in recipes

For a quick calorie count, you can refer to Chapter 16. But the foods you and your family eat aren't always as simple as the lists. With the help of those figures and the special ones for recipe quantities that begin on the next page, you can count the calories in a serving of anything from salad or stew to dessert. It's simple. Just look up the calories in each of the separate ingredients, total them, and divide by the suggested number of servings.

Here are the figures for Brown Stew:

2 pounds beef chuck	2,812
2 tablespoons fat	220
4 cups boiling water	0

Flavor boosters that don't cost calories
- 1 teaspoon lemon juice
- 1 teaspoon Worcestershire sauce
- 1 clove garlic
- 2 bay leaves
- Salt and pepper
- 1 tablespoon salt
- ½ teaspoon paprika

1 teaspoon sugar	16
6 carrots	126
1 pound small onions	172
Total:	3,346

Since the recipe is intended to serve **8** people, divide by **8**. This gives approximately **420** calories per serving.

Handy kitchen reference

Editor's note: 1 cup equals 8 fluid ounces, and there are 16 tablespoons in 1 cup.

Beverages

Milk:
    Condensed (sweetened),
        1 cup.................980
    Dry nonfat solids (skim),
        1 cup.................435
    Dry whole, 1 cup.........630
    Evaporated (unsweetened),
        1 cup.................345
    Fluid whole, 1 cup.......165
Carbonated water............0
Coffee, black...............0

Breadstuffs and grain

Bread crumbs, dry, 1 cup....340
Corn flakes, 1 cup...........95
Corn meal, yellow or white:
    Cooked, 1 cup...........120
    Dry, 1 cup..............525
Crackers:
    Graham, 4 small or
        2 medium..............55
    1 tablespoon cracker meal...45
Macaroni, cooked, 1 cup
    (1-in. pieces or elbow type).210
Noodles (containing egg),
    cooked, 1 cup...........110
Pancake mix:
    Buckwheat, 1 cup........430
    Wheat, 1 cup............470
Rolled oats, dry, 1 cup.....310
Rice, white, cooked, 1 cup ...200

Rye flour, light, 1 cup, sifted..285
Spaghetti, cooked, 1 cup.....220
Wheat flours:
    All-purpose or family flour,
        1 cup sifted...........400
    Cake or pastry flour,
        1 cup sifted...........365
    Whole, 1 cup............400
Wheat germ, 1 cup.........245
Wild rice, raw, 1 cup.......595

Candy

Candied or glace peel:
    Citron, 1 ounce...........90
    Lemon, orange, or grape-
        fruit peel, 1 ounce........90
Caramels, 1 ounce.........120
Chocolate, sweetened, milk,
    1 ounce.................145
Marshmallows, 1 ounce.......90
Peanut brittle, 1 ounce.......125

Cheese and eggs

American or Cheddar:
    1 cup grated.............445
Cream cheese, 1 tablespoon....55
Eggs:
    White, 1 egg white........15
    Whole, cooked in shell......75
    Yolk, 1 egg yolk..........60

Fats and oils

Butter, 1 cup.............1,605

Fats, cooking (vegetable):
1 cup 1,770
1 tablespoon 110
Lard:
1 cup 1,985
1 tablespoon 125
Margarine:
1 cup 1,615
1 tablespoon 100
Oils, salad or cooking:
1 cup 1,945
1 tablespoon 125
Peanut butter, 1 tablespoon . . . 90
Salad dressings:
Commercial, plain salad
dressing:
1 cup 900
1 tablespoon 60
French:
1 cup 945
1 tablespoon 60
Home-cooked, boiled:
1 cup 445
1 tablespoon 30
Mayonnaise:
1 cup 1,450
1 tablespoon 90

Fish

Haddock, cooked, fried,
1 pound 675
Halibut, broiled, 1 pound 825
Oysters, raw, 1 cup (13-19,
med. size) 200

Fruits and juices

Apples, 1 cup, cubed or sliced . . 85

Applesauce:
1 cup, sweetened 185
1 cup, unsweetened 100
Avocados:
1 cup ½-in. cubes 370
½ peeled (3½x3¼ in.
diam.) 280
Bananas, 1 cup sliced 135
Blackberries:
Canned, solids and liquid:
Syrup pack, 1 cup 215
Water pack, 1 cup 105
Raw, 1 cup 80
Blueberries:
Canned, solids and liquids:
Syrup pack, 1 cup 245
Water pack, 1 cup 90
Frozen, without sugar,
3 ounces 50
Raw, 1 cup 85
Cherries, red, sour, pitted,
canned, 1 cup 120
Dates, fresh, dried, and pitted,
1 cup 505
Fruit cocktail, 1 cup 180
Grapefruit:
Canned in syrup, solids and
liquid, 1 cup 180
Raw, 1 cup sections 75
Oranges, 1 cup sections 85
Pineapple, canned, syrup pack,
solids and liquid:
1 cup crushed 205
2 small or 1 large slice,
plus 2 tablespoons juice . . . 95
Frozen, 4 ounces 95
Raisins, dried, 1 cup 430
Raspberries:
Black, raw, 1 cup 100

Red, raw, 1 cup..........70
Frozen, 3 ounces..........85

Rhubarb, cooked, sugar
added, 1 cup............385

Strawberries:
Frozen, 3 ounces..........90
Raw, 1 cup..............55

Lemon or lime juice,
1 tablespoon..............5

Tomato juice, 1 cup.........50

Meat

Beef cuts, cooked:
Chuck, 1 pound with
bone...............1,140
Hamburger, 1 pound....1,655
Porterhouse, 1 pound
with bone...........1,270
Rib roast, 1 pound with
bone...............1,050
Round, 1 pound with bone..915
Rump, 1 pound with
bone...............1,175
Sirloin, 1 pound with
bone...............1,175

Beef, dried or chipped, 1 cup..335

Chicken:
Canned, boned, 3 ounces...170
Raw:
Broiler, ½ bird (8 ounces,
bone out)............330
Fryer:
1 breast (8 ounces,
bone out)..........210
1 leg (5 ounces, bone
out)...............160
Hen, stewing chicken (4
ounces, bone out).....340

Roaster (4 ounces, bone
out)................225

Lamb:
Leg roast, 1 pound with
bone.................980
Rib chop, 1 pound with
bone.................1,255
Shoulder roast, 1 pound,
with bone............1,160

Pork, fresh:
Ham, 1 pound with bone.1,430
Loin or chops, 1 pound
with bone...........1,150

Pork, cured:
Ham, smoked, cooked:
1 pound with bone....1,495
1 pound without bone..1,805

Veal, cooked:
Cutlet, 1 pound without
bone.................995
Shoulder roast, 1 pound
with bone.............760
Stew meat, 1 pound without
bone.................1,345

Nuts

Almonds, 1 cup.............850

Brazil nuts, 1 cup...........905

Cashew nuts, 1 ounce........165

Peanuts:
1 cup medium halves......805
1 tablespoon, chopped......50

Pecans:
1 cup halves..............750
1 tablespoon, chopped......50

Walnuts:
1 cup halves..............655
1 tablespoon, chopped......50

Soups

Bouillon, 1 cube............2

Consomme (11-ounce can)....26

Cream soup (11-ounce can)..280

Tomato (11-ounce can)......230

Sugars and syrups

Honey, 1 tablespoon..........60

Jams, marmalades, preserves,
1 tablespoon...............55

Jellies, 1 tablespoon.........50

Molasses:
1 cup..................825
1 tablespoon..............50

Syrup, table blends (chiefly
corn syrup):
1 cup..................940
1 tablespoon..............55

Sugars:
Brown:
1 cup firm-packed.......815
1 tablespoon............50
Granulated, cane or beet:
1 cup.................770
1 tablespoon............50
Powdered, 1 cup..........495

Vegetables

Beans:
Canned or baked:
Pork and molasses, 1 cup.325
Pork and tomato sauce,
1 cup...............295
Green, cooked, 1 cup......25
Lima, cooked, 1 cup......152
Red kidney, canned (or
cooked) solids and liquid,

1 cup.................230

Beets, 1 cup diced, cooked.....70

Cabbage, 1 cup, shredded
finely, raw...............25

Carrots, raw:
1 carrot (5½x1 in.).......20
1 cup grated.............45

Cauliflower, raw, 1 cup
flower buds..............25

Celery, bleached, raw:
1 large outer stalk (8 in.
long)..................5
1 cup diced..............20

Endive, raw, 1 pound........90

Escarole, raw, 1 pound......90

Lettuce:
1 head, compact..........70
1 head, loose-leaf.........30
2 large or 4 small leaves......7

Mung bean sprouts, 1 cup.....20

Mushrooms, canned, solids
and liquid, 1 cup.........30

Onions, raw, 1 tablespoon,
chopped.................5

Onions, young green, 6 small
without tops.............25

Parsley, 1 tablespoon, chopped..1

Peppers, green, 1 medium.....15

Pimientos, canned, 1 medium..10

Potatoes:
Boiled, 1 medium potato
(2½ in. diam.) or 1 cup
diced.................105
Mashed, milk added,
no butter, 1 cup........160

Potato chips, 10 medium (2
in. diam.) or 7 large (3
in. diam.)..............110

Pumpkin, canned, 1 cup......75

Tomatoes, canned or cooked,
   1 cup.................. 45

Miscellaneous

Chili sauce, 1 tablespoon......15

Chocolate, cooking:
   Sweetened, plain, 1 ounce..135
   Unsweetened, 1 ounce.....140

Chocolate syrup, 1 tablespoon..40

Cocoa, breakfast, plain, dry
   powder, 1 cup, stirred before
      measuring.............330

Coconut, dried, 1 cup.......345

Gelatin, dry:
   Dessert powder, 3-ounce
      package..............325

Plain, 1 tablespoon........35

Malted milk, dry powder,
   1 ounce..................115

Starch (corn), 1 tablespoon....30

Tapioca, dry, 1 tablespoon,
   granulated, quick-cooking...35

Tomato catsup:
   1 cup....................270
   1 tablespoon..............15

Tomato puree, canned, 1 cup. 90

Vinegar, 1 tablespoon.........2

White sauce, medium, 1 cup..430

Yeast:
   Compressed, baker's, 1
      ounce................25
   Dried, brewer's, 1
      tablespoon.............20

Chapter 8

When you're away

from home plate

A popular excuse for falling off the diet wagon is, "I'm always being invited out, and if I don't eat what my hostess serves, she'll never ask me to her home again." That alibi sounds like sweet reasonableness, but is as hollow as can be. You'd think that social success is measured by gastric capacity. To be sure, it isn't a very good friend-making idea to scan the festive dinner table with a glacial eye and remark, "I'm sorry, there's nothing here I can eat. I'm on a very strict diet." That sort of thing can be disturbing to a hostess who has slaved all afternoon. And what you've said isn't true. There's always something you can eat.

It may be hidden under drifting clouds of whipped cream, or swimming in a richly exotic sauce ("I practically *stole* it from the chef at a quaint little place in Paris"), but there's a reducing diet on every social dinner table. And you can pick it out very easily, too, after you have practiced a little. There are plenty of other things you can do to remove dieting as an obstacle between yourself and your hostess.

You can tell her in advance. A telephone call will prepare her for the worst—you can't eat pork, you love a raw apple for dessert, tussling with the paper pants on a lamb chop is more exercise than you're allowed. Whatever the stark necessities may be, she'd like to be forewarned.

You can leave things on your plate. Strangely, hardly a soul will notice. It isn't the calories on your plate but those in your stomach that count. Meat? Trim off fat, nudge off gravy with a sly sidling fork motion. You can invent a dozen other such tricks once you learn what calorie-rich foods to forgo. Don't feel guilty. Better let food go to waste than to waist.

You can take seconds ostentatiously. This is really high-class trickery. People will marvel how you stay so slim though you never stop eating. When the green beans come around the second time, really load your plate. Pile it high with broccoli, celery, spinach—there'll be at least one low- or lower-calorie item that you will recognize. With a mountain of fibrous foliage on your plate, there won't be room for gravied dumplings and other rich delicacies, and you can give the illusion of eating voraciously without actually doing so.

As artistry improves, the technique can be applied to the whole dinner. You become so fascinated by table talk

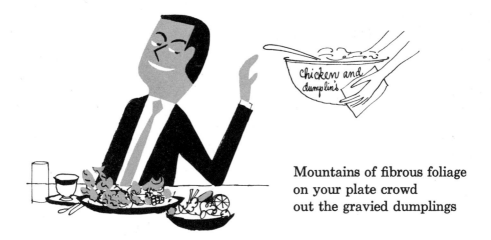

Mountains of fibrous foliage
on your plate crowd
out the gravied dumplings

that everyone else finishes before you do. And when the plates are whisked away, nobody realizes that you ate only the foods appropriate to your diet.

You can turn the spotlight away from diet. It's a very odd thing, but no one will know you are dieting unless you tell them. Go right ahead, eat a little less of rich foods—it's 10 to 1 nobody will even notice. This may sound as if you don't have to practice calculated trickery to circumvent your hostess. That's right. "My friends force so much food on me that I can't reduce" just doesn't stand up. Your fat is in *your* hands.

Reckoning with restaurants

Dining out in restaurants need not wreck a reducing program. Sometimes an eating place specializes in a particular delicacy, and when we're with a group we want to eat what everybody else is enjoying. Suppose the specialty is French-fried chicken. Remove the delicious outer crust. With a magnificent display of will power, leave it on your plate. The chicken itself is a splendid protein food. Occasionally, we may have to choose the lesser evil (calorifically evil) when there is limited variety.

But most of the time, the selection of a reducer's meal from the generous list on a restaurant menu is completely under our own control. Quite a few restaurants make a big point of listing low-calorie meals or foods for weight-conscious customers. You can find such foods on practically any menu, even though they aren't billboarded.

There's a handy, simple formula for assembling a fine reducer's meal from any restaurant menu you're likely to encounter. It goes like this:

Appetizer: Consomme or any clear soup (not creamed), melon, fresh-fruit cup, grapefruit or tomato juice.

Main course: Lean meat or fish. Cut away visible fat if any. Choose two vegetables, preferably one green and one yellow: asparagus, wax or green beans, broccoli, Brussels sprouts, cabbage, carrots, cauliflower, celery, cucumbers, greens, mushrooms, onions, rutabagas, sauerkraut, spinach, squash, tomatoes.

Salad: Lettuce, endive, Bibb lettuce, escarole, water cress, cabbage, tomatoes, aspic.

A chef's salad of crisp vegetables, chicken strips,

tongue, sliced hard-cooked egg, Roquefort or blue cheese, makes a good main-course lunch. Ask for tomato juice or lemon instead of a rich dressing.

Bread: Bread, rolls, and butter are often served before the waiter takes your order. A lot of unconscious nibbling can be done while you're waiting for the first course (or the waiter). Bread and rolls are fine foods, and reasonable amounts are allowed in all except very low-calorie reducing diets. Just remember your quota; pass up sweet rolls, cinnamon buns, etc. Your butter allowance may be one pat. Let the chilled pat soften on your plate, so it will spread more thinly and go farther.

Dessert: Raw, canned, or stewed fruit (you needn't eat all the syrupy juices), berries, melon, baked custard, a little cheese and crackers.

Beverage: Coffee or tea without cream or sugar, milk, or buttermilk.

Once in a while you may want to splurge with friends in some posh restaurant. If you feel that you are going to have to eat more heavily than you ought to, "save" an item allowed you in a previous meal of the day. Consume this food in the big meal later with a righteous feeling.

Lunch counters and cafeterias

There's nothing nutritionally horrible about a quick lunch of a beverage and a sandwich. It all depends on the ingredients. Certainly, a lunch of black coffee and a jelly sandwich makes a dietitian shudder. But a well-chosen sandwich can be a nourishing meal in itself. Enriched or whole-grain bread, a good protein filling, sliced meat, cheese, egg—with maybe some lettuce and sliced tomato —furnish separate courses.

Now add a glass of milk or buttermilk, and possibly a raw or stewed fruit for dessert, and you've done right well by your economy.

Soda-fountain counters, roadside lunchrooms, and cafeterias usually feature "short order" meals and sandwiches. So when you stop for nourishment on a motor trip, or order something sent up to the office from the drugstore downstairs, or inch forward in a cafeteria line, it's important to know what to order. It may help to remember that your stomach doesn't care whether proteins, carbohydrates, fats, minerals, or vitamins arrive from a sandwich or a salad or a beverage. Once you've followed and enjoyed the reducing meals in this book for a few days, you won't have much trouble recognizing many of the same foods when they reappear in the form of sandwiches.

Mainly, you'll want to keep as much *fat* out of sandwiches as possible. If the entire lunch is to be a sandwich, the calories furnished by the dressing and salad spreads and butter may not be excessive (of course, people who are not reducing need those calories).

Broiled hamburger is a safe choice. Generally it's placed on a bun that sops up a good deal of the fat juices. The result is delicious, but if you leave the juicy bread

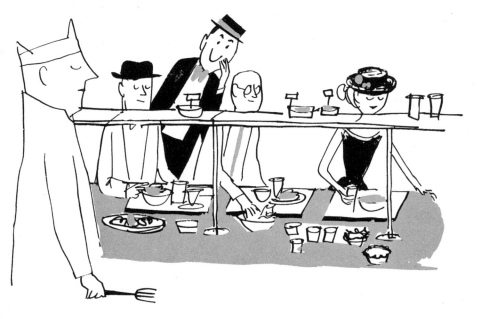

Cafeterias threaten with eye appeal. Protect yourself from an overloaded tray. Window shop before you choose your food

untouched, using a dry bun if you like, you will have escaped quite a few calories.

Cafeterias exert one subtle threat. They have eye-appeal—a delectable array of foods that tempt you as you march past. If people ahead and behind are jostling, you may snatch this or that food and wind up with a tray loaded with much more than you intended to eat. In a strange cafeteria, protect yourself by sauntering along outside the rail, just window-shopping. Then, when you get in line, you'll know what's coming.

Naturally the given "formulas" are not ironclad. They are merely intended to show you that a well-balanced and relatively low-calorie selection of foods can be made from almost any restaurant menu. You will see why the reducing diets in this book are built around foods that are common to *normal diets*. Your reducing diet is not a weird, exotic collection of "miracle" foods that no normal person would dream of following indefinitely. On the contrary, it's a framework for *permanent* good diet and good eating, too. So you shouldn't be in the least surprised to find many of the same foods served by your favorite restaurant, if you only look for them.

Chapter 9

Make use of

special foods

An increasingly popular class of products looms large in the food industry these days. They loom especially large in the eyes of folk who don't want to loom quite so large themselves. They are special dietetic foods, reduced in calories, designed to satisfy the reducer's sweet tooth without wrecking his diet. Nonnutritive, calorie-free sweetening agents are used instead of sugar. Some special foods use low-calorie ingredients to replace fats and oils in such things as salad dressings. Others use reduced-calorie recipes in preparing baked goods and cereals.

At least 200 different diet items of this nature are marketed by upwards of 60 specialized companies. The bill of fare includes canned fruits, fruit juices, jellies, marmalade, puddings, soft drinks, salad dressings, candies, soups, cake mixes, noodles, spaghetti, macaroni, bread, crackers, cookies, and the list continues to grow. If you wish to use some of these foods while you are reducing, or to help you stay reduced, chances are that you will find at least some of them on the shelf of your neighborhood food market. About 80 percent of supermarkets, the country over, have installed dietetic departments featuring low-calorie foods. When you are discussing your reducing plans with your doctor, it's a good idea to get his views about special dietetic foods you may want to use.

Many foods in this category are recognized for special dietetic purposes, but, disregarding calories, some contribute larger amounts of important nutrients to the diet than others. In general, the reducer can substitute a "diet pack" food made without added sugar, for the same food as ordinarily packed, and obtain natural food values without added calories. The main thing that bothers authorities is the possibility that nonreducers, who need their calories, may unwittingly buy and consume some special low-calorie food, never realizing that they have unintentionally deprived themselves of a calorie-cargo that isn't there. It's a good idea to read the label.

Frankly, the principal advantage of some special dietetic foods is convenience. "Diebetic" or water-pack canned fruits have been on the market for a good many years. Low-calorie jellies, puddings, marmalades, salad dressings are handy to have in ready-for-use commercial packages. There is, of course, almost no end of low-calorie foodstuffs that a dedicated housewife—dedicated to a slimmer waistline—can concoct in her own kitchen if she has a mind to. Sodium and calcium cyclamates are medically accepted sweeteners of no caloric value that serve as sugar substitutes in many recipes. You'll find recipes for homemade, low-calorie salad dressings on page 103.

Since there are innumerable brand names, special products, and formula variations, we can't hope to list each and every one of these dietetic low-calorie foods. Even if we could, the list would be outdated in a month, at the rate these new products are entering the field.

Other foods than the specially prepared diet-pack kinds may have special values in reducing diets.

Fresh fruits, such as oranges, tangerines, apples, pears, and peaches require neither added sugar nor artificial sweetening. Eaten out of hand or in salads with low-calorie lemon, vinegar, or other dressings, they are valuable and satisfying when you are cutting down on calories. Fresh vegetable greens in salads, fresh radishes, onions, and carrot sticks are further extenders of special diets.

Most of the foods in the following list will be familiar to you, and the more important ones can be purchased from almost any food market. Some of these foods furnish important nutrients, such as vitamins, minerals, and proteins in very generous amounts, and they can be used liberally in reducing and other diets. Others cannot be consumed in large quantities, but in reasonable amounts are good supplements for stepping up the quality of a diet. A few of the listed products are drugstore rather than food-store items, and are for somewhat special purposes, for which a physician may prescribe them.

Nonfat dry milk solids (dry skim milk) supplies all the protein, minerals, and vitamins (except vitamin A) of whole milk, at about half the calorie cost. Do not substitute for whole milk in diets that *need* more calories. Available at most food markets, it comes in powder form and can be used either as powder or liquid. To reliquefy, follow directions on the package. The powder can be mixed with other dry ingredients in baking.

Skim milk can be bought in liquid form from most dairies. It provides all the important nutrients of whole milk except vitamin A in amounts equal to whole milk, but only half the calories. Skim milk can be "made" at home from regular whole milk by pouring off the top cream (this cannot be done with homogenized milk, in which the fat particles are evenly suspended). Or skim milk can be reliquefied by mixing nonfat dry milk solids with water, as above.

Buttermilk has the same nutritive value as skim milk and can be substituted if skim milk is difficult to obtain, as in restaurants, or if you like it better.

Cottage cheese is sometimes called pot cheese or farmer's cheese. Practically all commercial cottage cheese is made from skim milk, with added moisture (about three-fourths of cottage-cheese volume is water). Cottage cheese contains a very high concentration of biologically complete protein and important milk minerals, with relatively few calories. One ounce of cottage cheese (25 calories) contains two-thirds as much protein as one cup of whole milk (165 calories). Remember, most cottage cheese is creamed, thereby adding a few extra calories.

Yogurt. The food value of yogurt is substantially the same as that of the whole milk from which it is made. The characteristic sour flavor, which many people find delicious, and the custardlike texture of yogurt come from cultures of microorganisms "seeded" into whole milk. These may induce some changes in the intestinal flora (bacterial population), but, as far as is known, do not make any detectable contributions to nutrition per se. Yogurt is an excellent whole-milk addition to the diet, and, with or without addition of various flavoring agents, makes a most agreeable dessert.

Fresh vegetable juices. These are prepared by pressing the juices out of leafy and fibrous vegetables of all imaginable varieties. The vitamin and mineral content of the juices shows great variation, partly because of the different content of various vegetables, and partly because of differences in efficiency of extraction. If fresh vegetable juices are used, they should be consumed promptly after extraction, for plant cells, when crushed and damaged, liberate enzymes that destroy ascorbic acid, perhaps other vitamins. Vegetable juices have alkalizing values. However, even the best pressed juices (unlike purées) contain only fractions of the nutrients present in the original vegetable. The residue from carrots, cabbage, celery, spinach, after pressing contains valuable nutrients as well as bulk that can help to satisfy appetite and furnish roughage to assist in intestinal functions.

Wheat germ is a portion (about 2 percent) of the wheat

kernel that is removed from flours by ordinary milling procedures. It is rich in protein and an excellent source of vitamins of the B complex. Its fat content is about seven times greater than that of wheat flour, and ordinarily no great amount can be consumed at one time. The flaked germ can be sprinkled over cereals, mixed with drinks, or added to biscuit doughs or similar recipes in modest amounts. It is a good source of vitamin E and has considerable iron. Wheat germ is a useful protein and vitamin supplement to diets deficient in these elements. It is a good food, but performs no astonishing miracles. Wheat germ runs to about 15 calories per tablespoon. A sensible use of wheat germ would be to restore it to the diet in quantity comparable to that lost in the milling of grain—perhaps a tablespoon or so daily.

Brewer's yeast. Dried brewer's yeast contains protein of excellent quality. The proportion of protein is higher than in many ordinary foods (about one-half protein, one-half carbohydrate). It is an excellent source of B vitamins. Baker's yeast has similar values; it is higher in some B vitamins (niacin, riboflavin) than brewer's yeast, lower in others (thiamin). Combinations of dried brewer's and baker's yeast are often found on the market in flaked, powdered, or tablet form. The amounts of dried yeast that the average person can consume are quite limited (some people suffer abdominal distress), and the product is probably best regarded as a useful vitamin supplement to inadequate diets. One tablespoonful of dried yeast contains about 20 calories.

Unflavored gelatin. This product, available at all food markets, contains no sugar and is almost pure protein. It's protein is incomplete. One essential amino acid (tryptophane) is lacking, but the other essential ones are present as well as many others that add to protein materials of the body. Unflavored gelatin gives a convenient way of increasing protein intake that is particularly important in reducing diets—to help satisfy appetite and to provide building blocks for repairing the wear and tear of tissues. Unflavored gelatin is obtainable in packages containing the product in envelopes. Each envelope contains 7 grams (equal to one-tenth the recommended daily protein intake of adults), equivalent to 28 calories. The powdered gelatin can be dissolved in drinks, used in hot or jellied soups, in molds or desserts.

Flavored gelatin dessert. Now on the market you may buy a popular gelatin dessert. Your choice of flavors, they are all low on calories. These add a gay color note to the reducer's diet.

Protein hydrolysates. These products are familiar to your doctor under their trade names. They contain amino acids in powdered or granular form and have important medical uses whenever a patient's protein intake must be increased promptly and considerably. Many doctors prescribe protein hydrolysates or concentrates as plus-factors in reducing diets. The object is to increase the safety, efficiency, and satisfaction of reducing diets for reasons that have been discussed elsewhere. These products provide protein in highly concentrated form; for instance, 2 heaping tablespoons of one of them will supply one-fourth of an adult's daily protein requirement. Your doctor will tell you about these preparations.

Bulk producers. A chemical substance known as methylcellulose has unique properties that have led some physicians to employ it as an appetite-suppressor in persons who complain that they are "always hungry" on reducing diets. Methylcellulose can be compressed into a small tablet, but in the presence of water it absorbs moisture and expands into a soft, bland, jellylike mass. Methylcellulose has been used as a laxative, to provide nonirritating intestinal "smoothage." It appeared that this smooth bulk fooled the stomach into thinking it was full —as indeed it probably was, but not with food, for methylcellulose is entirely inert and has no calories. Now the substance has had some acceptance as a drugless aid to reducing, an appetite-deceiver. One maker includes methylcellulose in a product that looks and tastes like graham crackers. Each wafer supplies 30 calories but, taken with a full glass of water or milk between meals or a half-hour before meals, swells up to considerable bulk that gives a sense of fullness. Your doctor will know about these preparations and can judge whether or not they may be desirable in your flight from the calorie. Remember that these products expand in the stomach into surprisingly large amounts of bulk, so go easy on quantity.

Chapter 10

Dieting
family style

Who said you have to cook for two—one meal for the reducer, an entirely different one for other members of the family who need more calories? It just isn't so. Not if your reducing meals, like the ones in this book, are modeled closely to the normal diet you should follow after your weight is down. Your reducing diet is concentrated good nutrition. The rest of the family (and you, too, after you've slimmed down) simply add other good foods to the basic reducing diet. It's easy, and it's cheaper, too, for family meals are built around foods the reducer uses.

If you doubt that it's as easy as we say it is, look at the meals for one day, on page 164. The meal is for both the reducer and for the folks who don't need to reduce. It's the same basic meal, except the additional foods for nonreducers are listed on the right. Of course, the additional foods do not have to be the ones listed. It is always a good idea, in "expanding" a reducing diet to increase its calories with foods of superior nutritive value:

This shows how you

can diet and eat

with your family

You eat this	*Add for the family*
BREAKFAST Shredded wheat biscuit Milk Sugar Blueberries Canadian bacon Coffee	Egg prepared any way they like Buttered toast Cream instead of milk on cereal
LUNCH Chicken salad Rye wafer Strawberry-pineapple cup Milk Iced tea	Roll and butter instead of rye wafer Cookies
DINNER Veal steak (braised) Mashed potatoes Coleslaw Peas and carrots Small graham cracker Fresh peaches Milk Coffee	Butter on peas and carrots Gravy Bread instead of graham cracker Fresh peach sundae

more enriched or whole-grain bread and cereals, butter and margarine, fruits, fruit juices, green and yellow vegetables, milk products. But there's plenty of room, for those who don't have to watch their calories, to include desserts and dressings and gravies and favorite dishes that are too rich for weight-watchers.

Cooking procedures need not be ruinously upset. For instance, in preparing certain vegetable dishes, take out one portion for the reducer before rich sauces and seasonings are added. If you're baking apples for dessert, bake one apple without sugar for the reducer. Special low-calorie salad dressings (see page 103) can be made-up in advance and kept on hand. The reducer uses them, the rest of the family takes regular dressings. If home-fried potatoes have to be prepared for someone who loves them, the reducer can substitute a slice of whole-grain bread as a rough nutritional equivalent. Many food accessories, such as thick gravy or hard sauce, are served in separate containers, and are easily avoided if will power holds out.

We have pointed out in Chapter 8 that there is a good reducing diet hidden in practically every meal that is served you. The opposite problem, of expanding a reducing diet into one that contains more calories, is very simply solved in actual practice. If the above suggestions seem too, too obvious—and maybe they are—they're made to persuade you that "I can't go on a reducing diet because I haven't time to prepare two separate meals" is a very feeble alibi.

At about age 50, the body's metabolism or "speed of

living" begins to slow down a bit. We don't rush and bustle and tear about quite so recklessly as adolescents who are spendthrifts of energy. This is one of the rewards of maturity. We can enjoy life at a more leisurely pace. Since we don't burn up quite so much energy, we don't need to take in quite so much either. Our need for calories decreases, slowly and imperceptibly. Experts have figured out that for every decade of life, after age 50, intake of food calories should be decreased from 3 to 5 percent below the levels that have been maintaining us at normal weight.

Obesity is not much of a problem to elderly people, for the grim reason that really fat folk seldom live to be old. More often, a man or woman who is well along in years becomes an object of family concern because of "poor appetite." The contrast between the amount of food that Grandma eats and the amount stowed away by a high-school boy can be pretty startling. Yet many a healthy, elderly woman can maintain herself on 1,500 calories a day, or an older man on 2,000 calories—either of which would constitute a reducing diet for many overweight young people.

Usually, older folk needn't be nagged at, and needn't nag themselves, because they don't eat enough. Caloric intake is probably adequate—of course, dietary needs may be modified by infirmities or chronic ailments, and special requirements, if any, can only be determined by the physician who is taking care of the general health of the elderly patient.

But, if quantity of food eaten by elderly people in gen-

Older people need...

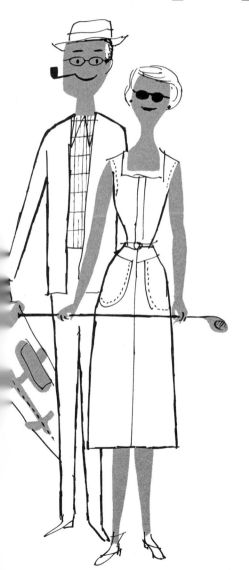

...fewer calories

...a diet relatively
low in fat

...naturally occurring
sugars and starches

...to avoid getting in
a food-rut—
eat a variety of foods

...more protein—
less carbohydrates
and fats

...a regular physical
checkup

eral good health is not seriously deficient, *quality* can be quite a different matter. When fewer calories are consumed, as needs decrease with age, it is all the more important that those calories be obtained from protective foods that give life to our years and vice versa. How can one plan a good, protective diet that is especially well suited to the needs of persons who are getting along in years? These general points are easy to remember:

It should be relatively low in fats (partly because fats play a probable part in hardening of the arteries, partly because liberal fat intake tends to lessen the amounts of protective foods that would otherwise be consumed on a relatively low-calorie diet).

Sugars and starches (carbohydrates) should be obtained from foods that are not highly concentrated or overrefined. Raw or cooked fruits, root and leafy vegetables, cereals and breads, contain naturally occurring carbohydrates that make fewer demands on sugar-regulating mechanisms of the body.

Intake of vitamins, minerals, and bulk is enhanced by eating a variety of the above and other foods.

A sedentary person needs as much protein as a very active person, but less fat and carbohydrate.

Do those specifications sound very much like the plan for a well-balanced reducing diet? So they are! If you are getting along in years, or if you prepare the meals for "old folks" who are living with the family, the 1,500-calorie meals in Chapter 7 are excellent for improving the eating habits of the elderly. Generous intake of essential nutrients is provided by the variety of foods allowed. An *additional* 500 or even 1,000 calories may be needed by many older persons who are quite active.

Sometimes, a physical ailment may dull the edge of appetite, or interfere with absorption of food. It is most important to have a health checkup by one's physician so that such conditions can be corrected. And he will advise the approximate number of calories necessary to sustain bodily vigor, if the patient's customary intake has been too low. Protective calories can easily be added to the 1,500-calorie menus by eating more bread and cereals, dairy products, fruits and vegetables—plus some delicacy that one particularly likes, that is eaten just for the fun of eating. Vitamin supplements and medical measures that the doctor will know about are often prescribed to counteract some of the changes brought by advancing years.

Habits, indifference, physical changes, often are responsible for poor nutrition in the elderly that is totally unnecessary. Deficiencies may arise if chewy foods are avoided because of ill-fitting dentures or sore gums. Steaks may be too difficult and important protein intake may suffer. However, there are many manageable sources of protein that are just as good or better than sirloin or porterhouse. Meats can be ground, chopped, stewed to softness. Cheese, cottage cheese, eggs, milk, unflavored gelatin, are fine protein foods that can be handled by practically any jaw that is still movable. Strained, pureed, or stewed fruits and vegetables can be used if ordinary forms are too tough for comfort.

Rigid food habits—such as an aversion to "rabbit

food" salads that grandpa considered unfit for he-men in his youth—may make one shun foods that are packed with good nutrition. Or the diet may become limited to a few foods that are perfectly good in themselves, but quite unable to supply the variety that is the basis of good nutrition. An elderly woman, living alone, may limit herself to one or two foods that are very simple to prepare and suffer from an unbalanced tea-and-toast diet. In the case of an elderly man and wife living together, the husband is a captive of his wife's food tastes; he eats—he'd better, anyhow—what's set before him.

Most of these saboteurs of good nutrition can be overcome if one is only convinced that it's worthwhile to make the effort.

Feeding the adolescent

Babies are generally well-nourished because mother is very conscientous about following the pediatrician's feeding directions. But as children grow older, they begin to escape to some extent from the family table and the watchfulness of a mother who is careful to prepare well-balanced meals. As a group, teen-agers are quite likely not to be eating what they should. A recent Cornell University survey of New York State youngsters found that half the teen-agers checked were not getting the nutrients recommended for good health. Worst backsliders from good diet were teen-age girls. These ill-fed youngsters were citizens of a state that ranks high nutritionally in the nation.

wrong | right

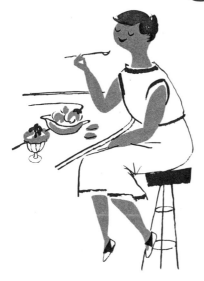

Eats snacks *first* . . .

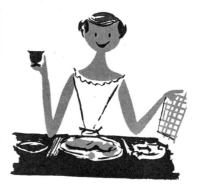

Eats MEAL first . . .

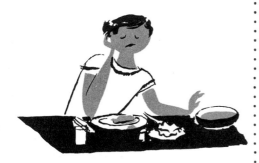

no room left for a
nutritious meal

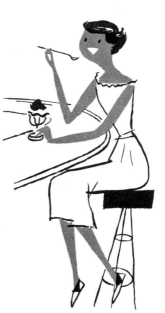

then eat sweets

Why do adolescents tend to be worse off nutritionally than younger brothers and sisters? Undoubtedly, some teen-age girls plunge into faddist reducing diets, or even well-balanced reducing diets, when they shouldn't reduce at all. The prime requisite to reducing, that excess body fat be present, has been stressed elsewhere in this book. Most adolescent girls go through an "awkward age" before the body matures into the pleasing proportions of the youthful feminine figure. There's a little too much here, and not enough there, before the curves come in the right places. At this stage, a heartsick young teen-ager may try to starve herself, or start on a magic diet or fast days or whatever, advised by some glamorous movie queen who has to stand broadside to cast a shadow. Or, on the other hand, the youngster may stuff herself with foods, especially all sorts of rich ones, to dull her feeling that she is ugly.

Mainly, the Cornell researchers concluded that the bad nutritional state of many adolescents is to be blamed on the fact that they have considerable freedom in choice of foods they eat, and do not choose wisely. Sweet snacks, eaten after school or too soon before dinner, can take the edge off appetite so a youngster is not hungry for the good full meal that mother puts on the plate.

What to do about it? Education in good nutrition, creating genuine liking for a wholesome variety of excellent foods, begins at home. Eating likes and dislikes are so much a matter of *habit* that the youngster who grows up in a home where a well-balanced diet is the rule is protected in his choices almost automatically. Pack his

Teen-agers should...

...be *sure* fat is present
before they reduce

...find a hobby if
they eat
because they're bored

...eat tempting confections
after they eat
necessary foods,
not in place of them

...eat fresh fruits
to stave off between-
meal starvation

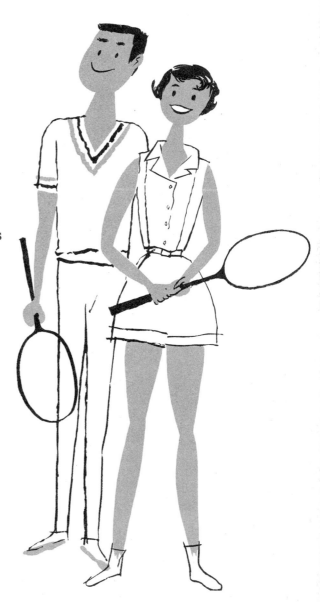

school lunch with nutritious sandwiches (for recipes, see page 106), milk, fruit for dessert.

If a good sandwich or meal is eaten first, then a tempting drink or confection when the crowd stops at the soda fountain can top it off, and many adolescents can use the extra calories to great advantage—provided they don't go overboard and use sweets as substitutes for important portions of their meals. Snacks are as natural as life to adolescents, and it's a good idea to revive the old custom of the family fruit bowl. Hungry youngsters snatch what's handy—a banana, apple, pear, orange, or peach sweetly fills an aching void and contributes important nutrients as well. Carrot and celery sticks, cheese, a bottle of milk, are fine to have on the front shelf of the refrigerator where a youngster stricken by mid-meal starvation will see 'em first.

A few things that take effort to chew should be included in every youngster's diet. Apart from nutritional values, foods that are coarse, tough, fibrous, crunchy, or stringy help the development of teeth, jaws, and gums. A normal bite, or proper contact of upper and lower teeth, is greatly assisted by chewing solid foods that help opposing teeth to grow into healthy relationships to each other.

If you need to gain weight

The forgotten person in these diet-conscious days is the too-thin person who wants and needs to *gain* weight. If the problem is not quite so common as overweight, it's just as distressing to those who are sick and tired of being

If you want to gain, eat 7 times a day

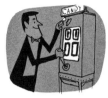

How to gain weight is a problem for some people. Try adding lots of foods like the following to the things you already like to eat.

Pick-me-up

Chocolate bar, peanuts, banana, hard candy kept in desk drawer, cupcakes

Breakfast

ham slice, egg scrambled in butter, coffeecake, cocoa

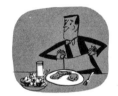

Dinner

buttered vegetables, mayonnaise or oil-and-vinegar dressing on salad, mints

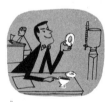

Coffee break

doughnut, sweet roll, plain or chocolate milk, cream and/or sugar in your coffee

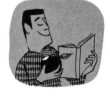

Munching

big apple, buttered popcorn, cheese and crackers, malt or milkshake, nuts

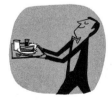

Lunch

grilled cheese sandwich, cream soup, potato chips

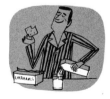

Bedtime

milk and graham crackers, cold fried chicken, sherbet

called bean poles. They may actually be sick and tired—
by which we mean that unexplained loss of weight and
appetite may be a symptom of some physical disorder. A
checkup by a physician is very important, because chronic weight loss may not be primarily a problem of diet, but
of some underlying ailment that demands skilled medical
treatment.

Most underweight people, however, have been that
way all their lives, and they yearn for a little extra padding to fend off the slings of fortune. Some have excellent
muscular development. They're the wiry, tireless, ener-
getic ones who can eat like a horse (a lean race horse) and
never put on fat. They burn energy usefully in pursuit of
their lean enterprises.

But other too-thin people tire easily, feel stuffed after
a few bites of food, think they're vaguely under par, and
suspect that they'd feel better if they could store away a
few calories where they'd show to advantage. Usually
they have tried to stuff themselves with eggnogs and
whipped-cream desserts and fried foods, only to find that
rich forced feedings make them so acutely miserable that
they just give up. The dinner-plate clue often identifies
such a person. He or she is very hungry, orders a good
meal, but appetite is satisfied so quickly that a very considerable proportion of the calories is left untouched on
the plate.

Why does such a person, who would love to eat like a
prizefighter, slow down and stop after a few mouthfuls?
The assimilative organs simply balk at a heavy load of
rich food *at one time*. But if food is taken in many small

meals, if one eats often but not too much at a time, a respectable total of calories can be consumed in the course of a day.

If simple weight gain is your problem, maybe you should try a six-or-seven-meal-a-day schedule. An eggnog between breakfast and lunch, a malted milk in midafternoon, a peanut-butter sandwich cached in your desk for furtive nibbling, cheese and crackers and milk before bedtime—choose the good protective foods that are the keystones of good diet. Fats and oils are desirable additions because of their heavy calorie cargo. Let comfort be your guide—don't try to eat so much fat at a time that you feel miserable. Wind up with any rich sweet that you enjoy, but don't eat sweets too soon before a meal or you may find your appetite gone. For that matter, space all your snacks so they don't spoil your appetite for regular meals.

In general, include the very foods that the overweight person can't have all he wants of: whole milk, cream, meat with fat, oily fishes, bacon, more butter and margarine, extra dabs of salad dressing, whipped-cream desserts, ice cream, gravy.

A very important aid to gaining weight has nothing to do with diet. In fact, many underweight people do not succeed in their attempts to gain weight by increasing their food intake until they learn this secret. It is *rest*. Relaxation. Many tense and intense too-slim people pour out prodigious amounts of energy, perhaps without realizing it. A slim person has more skin surface in relation to body mass than a fat one. Proportionately more calories escape from the "skin radiator." Even more important, the underweight person often has endless activities, jobs to do, committee meetings to attend, and conscientiousness or worry or responsibility may wind him or her up rather tightly inside so that a tense body wastes more energy than it ought to. Cutting responsibilities down to size, sloughing off some activities that are expendable, taking naps, lying down, giving one's self up to a chair for a few minutes when things are most hectic, early bedtime and plenty of sleep—such things are a wonderful help in persuading the calories one eats to stay around for a while.

Chapter 11

What minerals

do for you

You may not think that a few atoms of zinc and cobalt and magnesium are as essential to your life and every bit as glamorous as vitamins. But some trace minerals could as well be called metallic vitamins, since they function much as many vitamins do—as vital parts of enzymes that speed countless chemical processes that keep us alive. And some vitamins might reasonably be classed with minerals, since they would not *be* vitamins without minerals in their structure.

Minerals, like other nutrients, are ideally obtained by eating a wide variety of foods. But there are great variations in amounts of different minerals we need, as well as the amounts contained in common foods, and a little knowledge will serve you well in planning family meals.

What do minerals do for us? Some are important to body structures that keep us from collapsing. Others are parts of enzymes, chemical "spark plugs." The only environment in which we truly live is composed of mineral salts in solution. This is our internal environment, the fluids that bathe and nourish every cell. A need for minerals has been inseparable from life since its beginning.

The "Big Four" minerals are calcium, phosphorus, iron, and iodine. They are the ones most likely to be deficient in poorly planned diets, though they're no more important than other minerals that aren't so familiar. But remember, a variety of wholesome foods can supply all the minerals you need, including trace minerals.

Calcium

You use calcium to build and maintain the bony framework upon which the rest of you is hung. About 99 percent of your calcium is stored in your skeleton, representing approximately 2 percent of body weight. The other 1 percent that keeps circulating is fantastically important. If you prick your finger, calcium helps the blood to coagulate and plug up the injury.

Calcium is a powerful regulator of muscle contraction, and a minute amount of the mineral in the blood is necessary to keep your heart beating, for the heart is a hollow muscle. Calcium is a nerve-quieter, too, assisting in the transmission of nerve impulses through the body's communication system. Irritability increases when calcium decreases. Some kinds of muscle twitchings, cramps, and convulsions can be quickly relieved by making calcium salts available.

Your skeleton is not an inert mass of stony material. It's vitally alive. Most of the red blood corpuscles are manufactured in the marrow of long bones, and sharp little spikes of calcium project into these factories. If need arises, calcium can be stolen from living bone, withdrawn from the warehouse for distribution to tissues that need it desperately. The recommended daily intake of calcium by adults is 0.8 gram, less than 1 ounce per month. Infants, children, and adolescents, whose bones and teeth are still growing, need proportionately more calcium, and requirements increase during pregnancy and lactation.

Many authorities feel that calcium is the mineral most likely to be deficient in average diets. Perhaps most of us would do better to increase our calcium intake, and we might even add years to our lives by doing so. Dr. Henry C. Sherman, noted nutrition authority of Columbia University, made a famous study some years ago which proved that the lifespan of rats was increased 10 percent by diets containing abundant calcium. He also reported that signs of old age appear to be postponed in persons who get plenty of calcium as they grow up.

It is hard to get enough daily calcium unless milk or milk products are included in the diet. Not only whole fluid milk, but skim milk (which actually contains a trifle more calcium than equal amounts of whole milk), buttermilk, cheese, dry-milk solids, milk or milk solids used in baking, desserts, ice cream. Enriched flour and bread often contains added calcium as well as iron. Next best sources of calcium are green, leafy vegetables—kale, beets, greens, broccoli, collards, dandelion, etc. Dried beans and peas have fair calcium values. Meats don't contribute enough calcium to count for much, but fish and seafoods are fairly calcium-rich: mackerel, oysters, salmon, sardines, clams, and shrimp.

Unfortunately, the body does not necessarily utilize all the calcium that may be present in foods. In some leafy vegetables, calcium occurs in chemical forms that are partly or wholly unabsorbable. Even the calcium of milk is probably not utilized completely. Relatively large amounts of calcium are excreted from the body every day. Generous intake is best assured by eating a variety of foods that make for a well-balanced diet. Large doses of calcium salts, unless prescribed by a physician, can be hazardous and may upset the chemical checks and balances we live by. Excessive amounts of calcium, particularly if excessive amounts of vitamin D are also present, can lead to painful deposits, stone formation, hardening of soft tissues. And the amounts of calcium that we need and can profitably use are directly affected by phosphorus, a mineral with which calcium works very closely.

Phosphorus helps release energy

The old fallacy that fish is a specific "brain food" probably got started when it was found that the brain and nerves contain a good deal of phosphorus, and that fish are a good source of the element. Phosphorus compounds are certainly essential for nerve-cell activities, nerve-impulse transmission, and, one might guess, sparkling use of the brain. It is not unflattering to be called a fathead, provided the compliment is paid by a biologist who knows that phosphorus exists in the brain as a constituent part of the fat.

We couldn't lift a finger without phosphorus, which is essential for normal muscle activity and a vital element of compounds needed for utilization of energy. Phosphorus is part of the nuclear structure of every cell, necessary if cells are to divide and replace old cells that have worn out. Up to 80 percent of our phosphorus is used in building bones and teeth. Bone ash contains about half as much phosphorus as calcium.

Intake of phosphorus, as of calcium, is not just a matter of how much, but in what proportion. Calcium-phosphorus teamwork is so delicately proportioned that an excess of either mineral leads to excretion of the other.

Dietary deficiency of phosphorus is much less likely than calcium deficiency. Diets that contain meats can be presumed to have plenty of phosphorus. Milk is rich in phosphorus, in about the right proportion to calcium. Cereals, cheese, and eggs furnish good to excellent phosphorus quotas.

Iron puts steel into your blood

Iron puts steel into your blood. Each red blood cell contains a speck of iron. A red corpuscle is good for maybe 60,000 trips through your circulatory system before it gives up and quits. For replacement, you have to make literally millions of new red cells every *minute*. Each cell requires its speck of iron, and you'd think that your food would have to supply really stupendous amounts of ore. The listlessness, pallor, fatigue, and general tiredness of iron-deficiency anemia are quite enough to make us realize how iron stimulates our zest for living.

Yet a physician does not try to cure iron-deficiency anemia by merely advising that more iron-rich foods be eaten. It's all but impossible to overcome an established case of iron-deficiency anemia in any reasonable time by dietary means alone. But regular intake of foods that contain good iron is important, in order that we may have increased stores on hand if need arises.

Iron needs are increased by growth (that means children and adolescents), by pregnancy and lactation, and by blood losses. Aside from these conditions, there is hardly any evidence that a diet deficient in iron will produce iron-deficiency anemia. The reason is that the body hangs on like a bulldog to the iron it has. The iron of worn-out red cells is never wasted. It is used over and over again. In the ordinary sense, iron is not excreted from the body at all. But blood losses can carry iron out of the body. In men, and in women past the menopause, a true iron-deficiency anemia leads the physician to suspect that there is chronic, unsuspected blood loss, and he hunts for the cause which may be hemorrhoids, bleeding ulcer, or other conditions. It is futile to expect an iron-rich diet to do any good in such cases until the underlying cause has been corrected.

Monthly blood losses of women during their active reproductive years may increase their need for iron. Pregnancy and nursing increase iron needs, too—the baby is increasing its blood volume and supplies must come from the mother. Children need iron to make increasing quantities of blood. If there's a real deficiency, the doctor prescribes inorganic iron doses for prompt effectiveness and probably looks into dietary habits. (Milk is deficient in iron, and children who drink a couple of quarts a day, shunning other foods, may become anemic.)

Iron is widely distributed in animal and vegetable cells that are not excessively refined. Meat, eggs, colored vegetables (potatoes too!), whole-grain cereals, and iron-enriched white flour and bread are good sources. The amount of iron that is *assimilated* from foods is surprisingly small (but enough, for a' that), and one can by no means be confident that all the iron a food contains is going to somersault off into one's red blood cells. Spinach, for instance, has only a small proportion of its rich iron content in available form, and factors such as ascorbic acid and stomach acidity affect iron absorption. Fortunately, a well-balanced, varied diet supplies foods that furnish adequate iron almost automatically.

Iodine regulates body fires

Thyroid hormone is like a throttle that controls your body's speed. Body fires in people who have thyroid deficiencies burn low and smokily. They have a hard time keeping warm, skin is cold and clammy, hair coarse, physical and mental activity sluggish. People who have too much thyroid burn under forced draft, are always too hot, are big eaters but still grow thin, the heart races and eyes tend to pop, and mental and physical drives are quite intense. Most of us have approximately the right amount of thyroid hormone, so we're neither fireballs nor dullards. These very personal matters hinge upon minute amounts of one mineral, iodine, which constitutes 65 percent of the weight of thyroid hormone.

The body as a whole has only about one three-thousandth of an ounce of iodine and an equal amount in the thyroid gland—but what a difference it makes! The most common result of iodine deficiency is simple or endemic goiter, usually causing a visible swelling on the neck. When the thyroid runs short of iodine, it tries to make up for the lack by overworking itself and the usual result is neck-swelling or goiter. (There are other kinds of goiters, and all kinds call for medical diagnosis.) Seacoast dwellers run little danger of iodine deficiency, but in certain "goiter belt" areas of our country—the Great Lakes, Pacific Northwest, Rocky Mountain regions—soils and drinking water are poor in iodine. The simplest way to prevent *simple* goiter is to include iodized salt in the diet.

Foods supply variable but important amounts of iodine. Most reliable are seafoods, since iodine is relatively abundant in the oceans. Vegetables can be fairly good sources too, but everything depends upon iodine content of the soil on which they are grown, so comparative figures have no real meaning. Iodine is effective in prevention of simple goiter when given in any form and by any means. For reliability of iodine content, iodized salt ranks first, with seafoods a close second.

It's not possible to classify minerals as "most important" and "less important." They're all important, but some of those we talk about may sound strange and unfamiliar, and you may not know that you really can't live without them. Do not, however, feel that you have to fit exotic foods that are rich in trace minerals into your meals or take artificial supplements, or "balance" your diet with zinc and cobalt and so on. Deficiencies practically never occur in ordinary diets.

Sodium and chlorine = table salt

Life is impossible without sodium and chlorine, which is rather cheerful to know, since these two elements, properly married, constitute table salt. But there's no lack of these minerals in one's diet even though salt is not added to foods. Table salt, or sodium chloride, helps to maintain an acid-base balance and automatically keeps us "on the alkaline side." It is the most important mineral for maintaining osmotic pressure; that is, the forces which see to it that the right nutrients and materials get into and out of your cells. Salt is a factor in freer flow of saliva, digestive juices, and intestinal secretions.

It is hard to divorce sodium and chlorine, but the two minerals have some separate functions of their own. Chlorine is necessary for formation of hydrochloric acid in the stomach, an essential part of the digestive process. Sodium, not chlorine, is the element which, if taken in excessive amounts, causes water retention and a swollen condition of the body. Persons who are put on low-salt diets by their doctors are really on low-sodium diets, and the sodium from baking soda (sodium bicarbonate) is just as bad for them as table-salt sodium. It is possible to get too little sodium, if intake is too rigidly restricted by artificial diets, with symptoms that can be as bad as those caused by sodium excesses. A more common cause of sodium imbalance is the salt lost in perspiration. If sweating is very profuse, by reason of hard labor or hot weather or both, salt lost in perspiration is not replaced by ordinary drinking water. Painful muscle spasms known as "heat cramps" ensue if body fluids are diluted below a tolerable degree of saltiness. A little salt added to drinking water replaces the losses. However, the practice of adding a salt tablet to a glass of water just because the weather is warm is questionable unless a *great deal* of perspiration is actually being shed. "Heat cramps" generally occur under extreme conditions only, and most of us obtain plenty of salt from foods to make up the losses of ordinary hot-weather activity. Problems of sodium and chlorine intake are more likely to be of excess than deficiency as long as the salt cellar is on the table.

How to get your minerals

Quite clearly, it is humanly impossible to weigh and balance our daily intake of each and every essential mineral so that we feed exactly the needed amounts to our bodies. An excess of one mineral, or a deficiency of another, may throw the balances of both out of kilter. Excess table salt makes us lose potassium; too much calcium makes us excrete phosphorus, or vice versa; magnesium is antagonistic to calcium, and so on. To make matters more bewildering, some vital enzymes may function very well indeed by substituting any one of various metals in their structures, depending on what's handy. Harmonious *inter-relationships* between minerals are often more important than absolute quantities of particular single elements. Excesses of certain ones can upset applecarts we don't even know about.

Practically, it is not difficult to get a well-balanced intake of minerals if we don't become bewildered by trying to calculate specific nutrients—like the famous centipede that couldn't walk when it thought about which leg to move first. The simplest rule is to *include a wide variety of common foods in the diet* for automatic balance and protection. The iron that milk lacks is provided by eggs; vegetables often lack sodium but are rich in potassium; meats are good sources of phosphorus but not rich in calcium; and in a hundred other ways, one food balances another and no single food has all the nutrients we need in ideal proportions.

Mineral values for some foods must not be taken too literally, for mineral uptake from the soil depends on many factors. Acidity and alkalinity of soils, rainfall, and other factors modify the mineral uptake of plants. Again, a variety of foods from many sources is our best protection. Although they may have been grown many thousands of miles away from the part of the country in which you live, canned and frozen foods hang on to their mineral values superbly.

Cook your minerals kindly

Some vitamins, such as ascorbic acid, go to pieces when they're cooked, but most minerals can "take it" manfully when the heat is on. Some vital minerals may be drowned in cooking water and poured down the sink. Calcium, iron, phosphorus, and magnesium salts, for instance, dissolve quite readily in soft water.

To hoard minerals, then, cook with as little water as possible and use steam or pressure cookers if available.

The liquid contained in commercially canned foods holds water-soluble minerals and vitamins. *Use it*, if you want to get all the nutritive value. If it's more than you like to serve with a vegetable, pour it off, concentrate to one-half by boiling, add the vegetable, and heat just to boiling. Or use extra liquid for soups, sauces, or gravies.

Quick-freezing doesn't affect the mineral content of foods in the least. But kitchen carelessness can still play the villain. To retain all minerals, cook frozen foods according to directions—using a small amount of water for cooking, serving any excess liquid with the vegetable or using it for soups or sauces.

Chapter 12

If the doctor puts you on a special diet

Physicians prescribe special diets as part of the treatment of certain diseases. Foods that are extra-rich in particular substances may benefit some patients. Other patients may be put on diets that *forbid* those very same foods. Elements that help one patient are detrimental to another. Special-purpose diets, like medical prescriptions, must fit the needs of an individual. A bottle of cough medicine isn't of much use to a man who has a sprained ankle.

No one should start on a special-purpose diet without the orders and advice of a physician. One reason is that some special diets are deficient in vital nutrients and require vitamin or other supplements. Another reason is that even though a certain diet may be wonderful for a particular condition, there's no way of being sure that the condition exists unless the doctor says so. And he can't tell, either, until he has made a thorough checkup of the patient who needs custom-built advice.

In this chapter, we describe the more important special-purpose diets and indicate the conditions for which physicians prescribe them. No attempt is made to arrange the foods into daily meals, to indicate quantities or distribution, to point out deficiency dangers, except to remark upon the lack of wisdom of anyone who goes on a self-selected special diet because he hopes it's good for what ails him.

Sodium restricted (low-salt) diets

Low-salt diets are often prescribed for patients who have high blood pressure or heart and kidney ailments that lead to edema (retention of water in the tissues). Reduction of sodium, the element that "locks" water in the body, enables excess fluids to be excreted. Sodium, in combination with chlorine, is ordinary table salt, and low-salt diets are substantially the same as low-sodium diets. Low sodium intake tends to reduce the high blood pressures of many persons who have sustained hypertension. Effectiveness of the well-known rice-and-fruit juice diet in reducing high blood pressure is believed to be a result of its very low content of sodium.

Since sodium and chlorine are essential to life, no one should start on a low-sodium diet without medical advice. Serious conditions can arise from extreme sodium deficiency. By not using the salt cellar on foods, and by avoiding obviously salty foods such as smoked ham, average salt intake can be cut about in half. Sodium intake must be restricted more severely than that to be effective in cases where low-sodium diets are prescribed. The patient must be aware of possible sodium sources other than food: in drinking water, sodium bicarbonate (baking soda), food preservatives, drugs and medicines.

Low-sodium foods

Fresh vegetables: Asparagus, lima and string beans, broc-, coli, carrots, cabbage, Brussels sprouts, cauliflower, cucumbers, eggplant, onions, parsnips, potatoes (sweet or white), lettuce, tomatoes, mushrooms, green peppers, turnips, pumpkin, squash.

Eggs: Yolk only.

Fats: Unsalted (sweet) butter or margarine, vegetable oils.

Fruits and fruit juices: Apricots, grapes, pineapple, plums, oranges, grapefruit, apples, peaches, pears, figs (fresh or canned), all berries (fresh or canned), all fruit juices.

*Meat: Fresh or frozen meat or poultry, beef, lamb, veal, pork, chicken, or turkey; fresh, not frozen, fish.

†Milk: Not over 1 glass daily.

Sweets and desserts: Canned and fresh fruits, rice pudding, gelatin desserts, jellies, applesauce, apple butter,

---

*Meats are not low in sodium, but most patients are allowed one serving a day for protein values.

†Milk contains sodium and would be omitted from very strict low-sodium diets. Special low-sodium milk products are available, but other essential nutrients in milk are significantly reduced by low-sodium processing and the Council on Foods and Nutrition states that "such a product can no longer be called milk."

marmalade, maple syrup, sugar (check possible sodium preservatives in jellies, etc.).

Cereals: Wheat cereal, farina, oatmeal, buckwheat, rice, puffed rice, puffed wheat, macaroni.

Allowable spices and herbs to make low-salt foods more appetizing: Cloves, dry mustard, pepper, onion, vinegar, horse-radish, parsley, bay leaf, thyme, garlic, chives, basil, rosemary, marjoram, sage.

Go easy on these

All corned, pickled, smoked, or salted foods.

Dried meats, cold cuts, sausage, meat broth, stock, and meat extracts.

Sardines, herrings, anchovies, shellfish.

*Canned vegetables, meats, and soups.

†Frozen fish.

Egg white.

Cheese.

Beets, spinach, celery, greens, endive, corn.

Catsup, bouillon cubes, relishes.

Nuts.

Salted butter or margarine.

Dates, coconut, bananas, molasses.

‡Bread, biscuits, muffins, cakes, pies, cookies.

---

*Canned vegetables (unlike canned fruits) contain considerable sodium. Water-packed, "dietetic," low-sodium canned goods are packed by a number of manufacturers. Actual sodium content of such products is variable; uniform standards are not yet agreed on; check with your doctor.

†Some frozen fish is brine-processed. Many frozen vegetables are also brine-treated at one stage of the packing process.

‡Unless specially prepared without salt or egg white. Special low-salt breads are available in many localities.

Low-cholesterol (low-fat) diets

Cholesterol is a normal and necessary fatlike substance that circulates in our blood. In some people who have too much cholesterol or can't handle it properly, the substance may settle down in excessive patchy deposits inside the blood vessels and lead to a premature hardening of the arteries known as atherosclerosis. Favored targets for such deposits are the coronary arteries that supply blood to the heart muscle.

If these vessels become thickened and narrowed, like boiler pipes encrusted with scale, not enough blood gets to the heart when it works hard and the result is chest pain (angina pectoris). A coronary artery branch may be blocked, resulting in occlusion or thrombosis. Damaged arteries elsewhere in the body may give way. It is sad but true that we have no evidence that *anyone*, if he lives to 40 years, can survive without the development of arterio- or atherosclerosis in some degree. The discovery of vital facts about this process may well be the key to the place where the fountain of youth is kept.

Cholesterol, a suspect as a basic factor in the artery-hardening process, is the subject of a tremendous amount of research by medical scientists who are seeking ways of lessening the appalling toll of death and disablement charged to cardio-vascular diseases. One line of attack is to reduce the *dietary intake* of cholesterol, thus removing some of the raw materials out of which the deposits inside the arteries are built. However, the problem is complicated by the fact that the body (particularly the liver) manufactures cholesterol, whether or not the substance is obtained from one's diet. Many authorities believe that susceptible persons are somehow unable to metabolize cholesterol efficiently. And there is considerable evidence that the amount of cholesterol in the diet is less critical than *total fat* intake from foods.

Cholesterol levels of the blood usually drop when patients adhere to reducing diets that are naturally low in fats of all kinds. Dr. Ancel Keys of the Laboratory of Physiological Hygiene of the University of Minnesota has pointed out that the total fat content of American diets has been increasing for more than 40 years—from about 30 percent of calories consumed in 1909 to over 40 percent at present. "This," he says, "would more than account for the emergence of atherosclerosis to the dominance it now has in our mortality."

Cholesterol is present in animal fats but not in vegetable fats. Low-cholesterol diets principally exclude foods containing animal fats.

Foods low or lacking in cholesterol

Meat: Lean meats and poultry, all fat cut off; nonfat fish.
Cheese: Cottage cheese only.
Eggs: Egg white only.
Milk: Skim milk or buttermilk.
Cereals: All kinds.
Vegetables: All kinds.
Fruits: All kinds.
Desserts: Fruit, fruit juices, plain or flavored gelatin,

water ice, cornstarch puddings, meringues.

Soups: Consomme, bouillon, fat-free vegetable soup.

Beverages: Tea, coffee, carbonated drinks, juices.

Sweets: Sugar, jelly, jam, honey, molasses, hard sugar candy, maple syrup.

Fats: Olive oil, corn oil, peanut oil, other vegetable oils.

Go easy on these

All foods prepared with butter, cream, whole milk, lard, bacon grease, or other animal fats, including fried foods, potato chips, doughnuts, etc., unless vegetable fats are used.

Fatty meats, glandular meats: liver, brain, kidney, sweetbreads.

Egg yolk.

Whole milk, cream, butter, whipped cream.

Cream sauces, cream soups, gravies.

Foods made with eggs or animal-fat shortenings: pastry, cakes, rich desserts, ice cream.

Bulk (high-residue) diet

A certain amount of bulky material in the intestines is a necessary stimulus of normal bowel activity. Also important is the consistency (fluidity) of the material. High-bulk diets are often prescribed for correction of chronic constipation, in addition to other medical measures. Meat, fish, eggs, milk, cheese, and other concentrated foods that leave little residue are important for *balanced* diet. If the rest of the diet is largely starch, sugar, pastry, and candy, bulk may be insufficient. Intestinal bulk may not be of proper consistency if intake of fluids and fat is inadequate. Bulk diets for constipation stress fruits, liquids, fats, high-residue vegetables, and coarse cereals.

Bulk-diet foods

Fruits: Oranges, grapefruit, bananas, figs, apricots, cherries, peaches, apples, pears.

Dried fruits: Raisins, figs, prunes, apricots, others (good to stew, eat with breakfast foods and milk or cream).

Fruit juices: All kinds; do not supply bulk, like the pulp of fruits eaten whole, but are good source of liquids; and organic acids have mild laxative effect.

Cereals: Whole-grain kinds: oatmeal, puffed wheat, shredded wheat, *bran, etc.

Fats: Butter, margarine, cream, salad dressings, oils.

Bread, muffins, etc.: Coarser kinds; whole wheat, cracked wheat, rye, bran muffins, etc.

Vegetables: Leafy vegetables are slightly more effective bulk producers than others (use in salads) but all are good; serve some raw, others cooked. Frozen, canned, or fresh vegetables from the following list are in season all the time: Asparagus, string beans, broccoli, Brussels sprouts, cabbage, carrots, cauliflower, corn, eggplant, kohlrabi, lima beans, mushrooms, okra, onions, parsnips, green peas, peppers, potatoes, pumpkin, rhubarb, sauerkraut, spinach,

*Coarse foods may irritate some sensitive colons.

squash, Swiss chard, celery, endive, radishes, tomatoes, water cress.

Desserts: Ices, fruit, fruit whips, gelatin desserts.

Soups and beverages assist fluid intake.

Go easy on these

Highly refined cereals, fried greasy foods, macaroni, spaghetti, pastries.

Bland (ulcer) diets

Bland, nonirritating, acid-absorbing foods are generally prescribed for peptic ulcer patients and others who have inflammatory disorders of the stomach. Patients must, of course, be under careful medical supervision. The following list merely gives foods that are soft, smooth, free of rough fibers and seeds, and unlikely to cause chemical irritation or increased secretion of acid juices in the stomach.

Bland foods

Fruits: Remove skin, strain to remove coarse fibers if present. Raw ripe banana, ripe pear, cooked or canned apples, apricots, cherries, peaches, pears, prunes.

Fruit juices: Strain and dilute with equal parts of water.

Cereals: Refined wheat, corn, rice, dry breakfast cereals, cooked cereals, oatmeal, farina, macaroni, spaghetti, noodles.

Bread: Enriched white, toast, crackers.

Milk: Whole milk, skim milk.

Fats: Butter, margarine, cream.

Eggs: Soft-boiled, poached, souffle, or baked omelet.

Cheese: Cottage cheese or cream cheese.

Meat: Scraped or tender beef, lean meat, chicken, lamb, liver.

Fish: Fresh fish, canned tuna or salmon.

Vegetables: Potatoes (baked, boiled, mashed, creamed), cooked or pureed asparagus, beets, carrots, peas, pumpkin, spinach, squash, string beans.

Desserts: Gelatin, custards, ice cream, ices, tapioca, rice pudding, prune whip, angel-food or sponge cake, plain sugar cookies.

Beverages: Weak tea, milk.

Soups: Creamed soups of allowed vegetables.

Go easy on these

Coarse cereals, bran, breads made of scratchy grains, carbonated drinks, coffee, pork, veal, broth, bouillon, meat extracts, chili, highly spiced soups and meats, fried or greasy foods, gravy, raw fruits (other than those allowed), raw vegetables, nuts, pickles.

Acid-forming and alkali-forming foods

"Acidosis" is not a word for excess stomach acidity,

but for a *lessened* alkalinity of the blood. The blood does not become acid during life; it is *more* or *less* alkaline. In the treatment of some conditions, a strongly acid-forming diet may be desirable. For other ailments, an alkaline-forming diet may be prescribed.

The matter of acid-alkaline balance is beautifully taken care of by ordinary balanced diet. Vegetables and fruits are predominantly basic (alkali-forming). Cereals, meats, poultry, and fish are predominantly acid-forming. Unless we're seriously sick, we needn't worry about fussing with our diets to stay "on the alkaline side." Acid- or alkali-forming properties of foods do not depend upon acids in the foods themselves, but in the nature of the "ash" they leave when metabolized in the body. Fruits are mildly or strongly acid when eaten, but with very few exceptions their ultimate effect is an alkalinizing one.

Acid-forming foods

Barley	Goose	Pork
Beef	Haddock	Rice
Bread	Kidney	Rye
Cheese	Lentils	Sardines
Chicken	Liver	Shrimp
Corn	Lobster	Turkey
Crabs	Macaroni	Veal
Eggs	Mutton	Walnuts
Fish	Oatmeal	Wheat
Flour	Peanuts	

Alkali-forming foods

Apples	Currants	Pears
Apricots	Dates	Pineapple
Bananas	Eggplant	Potatoes
Beans	Figs	Pumpkins
Beets	Gooseberries	Raisins
Brazil nuts	Grapefruit	Raspberries
Broccoli	Grapes	Rhubarb
Brussels sprouts	Kale	Rutabaga
Cabbage	Kohlrabi	Spinach
Cantaloupe	Lemons	Squash
Carrots	Lettuce	Strawberries
Cauliflower	Milk	Sweet potatoes
Celery	Mushrooms	Tomatoes
Cherries	Oranges	Turnips
Coconut	Parsnips	Watermelon
Cucumbers	Peaches	

Neutral foods

Sugar	Lard	Cornstarch
Butter	Oil	Tapioca
Margarine		

Chapter 13

Don't overlook
calories in alcohol

Alcohol calories are peculiar, as some people have noticed. We are not here concerned with the social peculiarities of alcohol, but with its physiological behavior. Many essential nutrients are classified as alcohols (vitamin E, for instance). This discussion deals with ethyl or beverage alcohol, the kind that has been consumed by man since some ancient ancestor swallowed a spirited sample of cereals or fruits that had fermented accidentally through some carelessness of stone-age housekeeping.

One peculiarity of alcohol is that it is a depressant, not a stimulant as it often seems to be. It lifts the lid on inhibitions, depresses the central nervous system from the top down—that is, it first inhibits the more recently acquired higher functions of the brain, and gradually works down the evolutionary scale, so that activities essential to life, such as heart action, are depressed last of all. A modest amount of alcohol may therefore produce a reasonable facsimile of stimulation. But it is actually a fairly potent anesthetic, and indeed possesses the same carbon, hydrogen, and oxygen atoms as methyl ether, in slightly different arrangement.

Another peculiarity of alcohol is that the body has no way of storing its calories. Alcohol can be absorbed directly from the stomach without digestion. A very small proportion of alcohol calories is eliminated through breath and urine. But nearly all the alcohol a person consumes has to be burned and gotten rid of promptly. The body cannot store alcohol calories in the form of fat. It would seem that a person on a reducing diet, who wants to burn calories, could ignore alcohol intake. The catch is that although alcohol calories have to be oxidized promptly by the body, the calories of other foods are *not* burned to the extent they otherwise would be. If total caloric intake, including alcohol, is in excess of body needs, calories from foods will be stored as fat in amounts to make up for alcohol calories that are immediately burned.

The practical result is that the calories of alcohol have to be counted in a reducing diet, or any diet, just as if they came from ordinary foods. Other subtle effects of alcohol must be reckoned with too. It gives appetite a boost and at the same time anesthetizes inhibitions that give one strength to say no to food temptations. *Foods should never be subtracted from a reducing diet to make room for alcohol calories.* A carefully balanced low-calorie diet is designed to take care of nutritional needs; omission of important foods means that something essential is sacrificed. Alcohol calories, if consumed, should be counted as additions to a reducing diet. The effect will be to slow the diet's "reducing speed." Thus, a 1,000-calorie reducing diet, to which 2 ounces of 100-proof whiskey is added, will become a 1,200-calorie diet.

It is simple to count the alcohol calories of distilled liquors taken "straight," with no additions other than water, ice, or club soda. Whiskey, rum, gin, brandies, and similar liquors are sold by "proof"—100-proof, 86-proof, are common strengths. The amount of alcohol in the liquor is *one-half* the proof. Thus, 100-proof liquor is one-half alcohol. Alcohol contains 200 calories per ounce.

It is easier to figure the calorie values of proof liquors by the ounce, to simplify the arithmetic calculations of "jiggers" that may hold 1 ounce, or $1\frac{1}{4}$ or $1\frac{1}{2}$ ounces. Here is the formula:

1 ounce of 100-proof liquor = 100 calories.
1 ounce of 86-proof liquor = 86 calories.

In short, figured by the ounce of *liquor*, the calorie count is the same as the proof.

Other beverages are not so easy to figure, because the alcoholic content is expressed in percentages, or because sugars and other ingredients add calories in addition to alcohol. Mixed drinks such as cocktails, Collinses, toddies, vary considerably according to the proportions of ingredients used by the mixer. Dry wines contain fewer calories than sweet or fortified wines (the latter contain a little added alcohol plus the amount that naturally occurs during the winemaking process). Ordinary beers of the same alcoholic strength (average, 4 to 4½ percent), are substantially identical in calorie value and insignificant differences of other constituents make no practical difference to the waistline of the consumer.

The following table of alcohol calories of familiar liquors, wines, malt beverages, and mixed drinks, gives values as accurate as it is possible to obtain by analyses of average and representative samples. It should be remembered that differences of 10 or 20 calories between one drink or another are far too slight to have any significant meaning to the consumer.

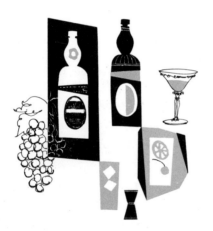

Table of alcohol calories

Wines,* per wine glass (3.2 ounces)

	Calories
Champagne, dry	90
Champagne, sweet	120

Fortified or dessert wines:
  Catawba. 140
  Muscatel. 165
  Port. 165
  Sherry. 140
  Vermouth, French. 110
  Vermouth, Italian. 175

Madeira. 110

Table wines, domestic:
  Burgundy, Chablis, Chianti, Claret, Reisling,
    Rhine, Zinfandel. 75

Sauterne, California. 90

Sauterne and Bordeaux, French. 80

Wines of the same type, for example, sherry or champagne, vary in sweetness. "Dry" or nonsweet wines usually contain fewer calories than sweet wines of the same type.

Distilled liquors, per 1½-ounce jigger (but jigger size will vary with the host)

Whiskies: rye, bourbon, Scotch, Irish; brandy; gin; rum; vodka

One serving 100-proof liquor. 150

One serving 86-proof liquor. 129

Highball with plain or carbonated water:
  100-proof liquor. 150
  86-proof liquor. 129

Highball with ginger ale:

100-proof liquor 180
86-proof liquor 160

Liqueurs, cordials, per cordial glass, ⅔ ounce

Benedictine, chartreuse, curacao, Cointreau, creme
de menthe, creme de cacao, sloe gin, maraschino,
etc., ... 75

Malt liquors, per glass (7–7½ ounces)

Ale 100

Beer (lager, Pilsener, bottle, or draught)* 100

Bock beer 135

3.2 beer 80

Porter, stout 150

Average 4 percent alcohol

Mixed drinks

Composition of mixed drinks is limited only by the in-
genuity, intent, and resources of the mixer. Proportions
of ingredients, amounts of sugar, fruits, syrups, juices,
and creams, and dilution by melting ice cubes, cannot
be calculated to the last fraction of a calorie for any
given, or purchased, drink as it is actually consumed.
But for all practical purposes, the following values are
entirely adequate for estimating caloric intake.

Cocktails, per cocktail glass (3 ounces)

Champagne (sugar, bitters, lemon peel)...........150

Dry Martini....................................150

Dry Manhattan.................................150

Old-fashioned (sugar, bitters, fruit)..............200

Regular Manhattan (Italian vermouth)...........175

Rum-base cocktails (Daiquiri, Bacardi, etc.—with
    sugar, syrups, citrus juice).....................175

Sweet cocktails (containing liqueurs, grenadine,
    sugar, cream, syrups, juices)—better count......200

Sweet Martini (with Italian vermouth)...........175

Tall drinks per glass about (7 ounces)

Collins—rum, gin, or whiskey base, with fruit
    juices and sugar, carbonated water............225

Eggnogs, flips, Tom and Jerry—distilled liquors
    with eggs, milk, sugar, cream, in varying pro-
    portions; for average serving, small cup of about
    4 ounces, better allow.......................250

Fizzes—brandy, gin, sloe gin base, lemon juice,
    sugar, carbonated water.....................225

Rickeys—gin, sloe gin, lime juice, and carbonated
    water.....................................175

Miscellaneous (for punctilious mixers who want to calculate separate ingredients of their favorite formulas)

Bitters, 1 teaspoon............................10

Cherry juice, 1 teaspoon........................7

Syrups—grenadine, raspberry, simple syrups,
   per ounce....................................75

For fruits, juices, cream, eggs, etc., consult general calorie table, page 237.

Note: Figures are averages, as accurate as it is possible to obtain, considering the variation in composition of many alcoholic liquors. Beers, wines, liqueurs, and many mixed drinks contain varying amounts of carbohydrate calories in addition to those from alcohol.

Chapter 14

All about

vitamins

Why do you need vitamins? If you knew all the answers to that question, scientists would be pounding at your door, begging to be let in on the secret. For, despite years of intensive study, scientists do not yet understand the complete functions of a single, solitary vitamin.

We may say that we need vitamins to prevent scurvy or rickets, or, if we want to sound wise, to prevent xeroph-thalmia or beriberi. We'd be right, too. But we'd be telling a pitifully small part of the story of those power-packed food factors we call vitamins.

In the early days of vitamins, they were viewed as things that make us sick if we *don't* get them. For instance, if you don't get ascorbic acid, you do get scurvy. Trouble is, researchers keep on discovering new facts about ascorbic acid. This increases their ignorance, for each new fact generally hints that other tantalizing facts are still hidden in the shadows. It is known that ascorbic acid is somehow important to our adrenal glands and their hormone output, that the vitamin plays a role in blood formation, connective-tissue growth, wound healing, and doubtless for reasons the experts haven't thought of yet.

The story is the same with other vitamins—there's a great deal yet to be learned about them. Fortunately, it isn't necessary to understand the chemical activities of vitamins in order to enjoy their benefits. But you may have a natural curiosity about these powerful little things that you swallow invisibly with your food each day. We'll try to satisfy that curiosity, to help you understand what vitamins can do for you, and, just as important, what they can't do.

What is a vitamin?

"I'm glad you asked that question," says the expert on a quiz show as he stalls for time, groping for a satisfactory answer. That's something like the predicament of experts who have great difficulty in defining vitamins as a group.

Vitamins have no common chemical structure that identifies them as vitamins. They may be acids or alcohols or other compounds, as different from each other as table salt and aspirin. They occur in foods, but vitamins are not foods in the ordinary sense. They do not furnish energy or build tissues. You'd soon starve to death if you ate nothing but vitamins. No amount of vitamins can change a thoroughly bad diet into a good one.

About the only way to be sure a vitamin is a vitamin is

to study its activities in living bodies, including our own. Every living thing, down to the tiniest germ, depends for its very life upon a wonderful group of substances known as biocatalysts. A catalyst is a substance which, by its mere presence, sparks a specific chemical reaction that couldn't occur without it.

You digest a meal with ease (and no little pleasure, if you are overweight) because digestive enzymes do most of the work of splitting food elements into the right chemical shapes for our use. Without such enzymes, it might take you 30 years to digest your dinner, and by then it wouldn't matter. Enzymes are catalysts of incredible power. One pound of pepsin, a stomach enzyme, could digest 30 tons of meat in a couple of hours. We have hundreds and hundreds of specific enzyme systems, each responsible for a chemical activity essential to our cells, which is to say, to life itself.

Vitamins seem to belong in this great category of biocatalysts, and many hormones, too. Many vitamins are known to be coenzymes, or essential parts of enzymes. We can now attempt to tell you what a vitamin *is*. It is a chemical substance of exactly the right make-up to bring proper groups of molecules together, so those molecules can exchange particles and produce a new substance necessary for some function of the body.

The vitamin is a catalyst, something like a clergyman, without whom a couple can't get married. The clergyman expedites the marriage, but is not a part of it; he can be "used" over and over again to perform other wedding ceremonies. Similarly, vitamins are not consumed in significant amounts by the processes they facilitate. That is why minute quantities of vitamins, regularly replenished, are quite adequate for the needs of normally healthy persons.

While we need more of some vitamins than of others, the quantities are still small. The amount of vitamin B_{12} that keeps a pernicious anemia victim in good health is one microgram daily. At that rate, a mere ounce of the vitamin would last you more than 500,000 years.

What vitamins do for you

Vitamins are regulators concerned with the release of energy and its utilization by the cells of our bodies. A pretty dull statement? Yes—but it becomes exciting when we turn the spotlight on you instead of your chemistry.

Most of the benefits that vitamins work for us are not nearly so dramatic as the cure of rickets or scurvy. Chemical processes of life are not direct and isolated, like the production of rust on an iron nail. They are interrelated chain reactions, great cycles of activity, in which molecules go through dozens or scores of successive changes until a final product is achieved. A vitamin may be necessary for only one step in such a cycle, but, if it isn't there, a link is missing and the chain is broken.

Symptoms of acute vitamin deficiencies are fairly obvious to the physician. Obscure effects are not so apparent.

Chances are you'll never have any of the extreme vitamin deficiency diseases. But you will feel fine, or not so fine, depending on what you eat.

Good health means more than just not being sick. It means you feel up and at 'em! Give yourself a more than adequate vitamin supply. Eat a wide variety of foods every day and you'll be more than likely to include all the kinds of vitamins you need. By not getting into a food rut, you can make already good nutrition better.

The following list of vitamins tells what scientists know or suspect (up to now) that vitamins do for you.

Vitamin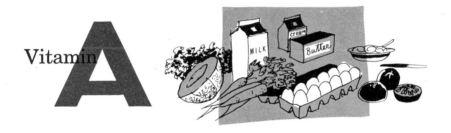

Vitamin A. Needed for growth of bones and teeth, for normal skin and mucous membranes, for seeing in dim light. (A theater is dark when you grope for a seat; soon the dimness is less and you can see quite clearly—vitamin A at work!) Deficiency symptoms: night blindness, dry skin, eruptions which resemble gooseflesh but do not disappear when rubbed, dryness of the eyes. Your liver can store enough vitamin A to last a long time, perhaps a year. Dietary deficiency of vitamin A is uncommon, but infants may need supplements before they begin to eat vegetables and egg yolk. Mineral oil and disturbed fat digestion may impair absorption of vitamin A.

Vitamin **B**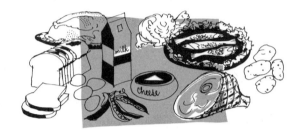

The B vitamins (B complex). Originally, vitamin B was thought to be a single substance. Now it is known to be a large family of vitamins, soluble in water, which have no chemical relationship to each other but are often found together in foods. Chemists classify the B vitamins in two main groups: one group is important to the release of energy from food, the other to formation of red blood cells.

Niacin. Necessary part of enzymes concerned with oxidation in our body cells; continued deficiency causes pellagra. Deficiency symptoms: red, burning tongue, insomnia, loss of appetite, irritability, vague burning sensations, numbness, skin lesions resembling sunburn, turning brown and scaly as disease progresses.

Riboflavin. Needed as part of vital enzymes; exactly how they work in the body is unknown. Deficiency symptoms: tiny blood vessels intrude into cornea (transparent window of the eye), lips redder than usual, whitened, fissured skin at corners of mouth, magenta-colored pebbly tongue, dermatitis about nose, cheeks, and chin.

Thiamin (vitamin B₁). Once called the "nerve vitamin" (and, by some careless enthusiasts, the "pep vitamin" supposed to load you with zest), thiamin is as important to normal function of heart, blood vessels, and digestive tract as it is to the nervous system. Acute deficiency, rarely seen in this country, leads to beriberi, a disease marked by congestive heart failure, neuritis, paralysis, and muscle atrophy. Milder, chronic deficiency is hard to diagnose because symptoms act like "personality complaints"— fatigue, dizziness, headache, irritability, poor concentration and memory. Food faddism, alcoholism, poorly prepared foods, may reduce dietary intake of thiamin.

Vitamin B₆. Marked deficiency of this vitamin may result in convulsions in babies. Ordinary pasteurized or evaporated milk contains an abundance of vitamin B_6— sufficient to prevent the occurrence of these symptoms.

Vitamin B₁₂. Essential to red blood cell formation, the most severe form of vitamin B_{12} deficiency is seen in pernicious anemia. Strangely, the pernicious anemia victim, like the rest of us, usually gets plenty of vitamin B_{12} from food. What the victim presumably lacks is not the vitamin, but an unknown substance secreted by normal stomachs, called intrinsic factor, which in some way "pushes" B_{12} through the intestinal walls into the body. At present it appears that lack of infinitesimal amounts of intrinsic factor thus blocks a cycle of chemical processes indispensable to health, just as absence of vitamins may block other cycles.

Vitamin C

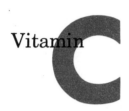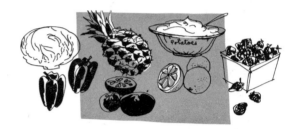

Ascorbic acid (vitamin C). This vitamin seems necessary for adrenal-gland functions, for use of some protein food elements, for absorption of food iron, for formation of long-chain protein molecules (collagen) that form framework of connective tissue, bone, dentine of the teeth. Severe deficiency causes scurvy, now relatively rare, except in some children under a year old. Mild scurvy in adults is not easy to diagnose. Suggestive signs may be pinpoint hemorrhages under skin, inflamed gums, loosened teeth, weakness, irritability, vague pains, slow healing of cuts and wounds. Daily supplies of ascorbic acid are necessary; diets lacking fresh fruits and vegetables suggest possible deficiency.

Vitamin D. It is necessary for proper use of calcium and phosphorus in blood, for bone formation; there is a possible relationship to pituitary, thyroid, and parathyroid glands. Deficiency results in loss of calcium and phosphorous, one of the direct causes of rickets in infants. It is most important to infants and growing children who need vitamin D supplements during growth. Most adults make enough vitamin D from the action of sunlight upon substances in their skin. Those habitually shielded from sunshine may need supplements.

Vitamin E. Most of the medical uses of this vitamin are frankly experimental, with generally disappointing results. Human requirements are unknown and there are no well-established symptoms of deficiency.

Vitamin K. Essential for making substances that enable blood to clot. Deficiency increases bleeding tendencies, but dietary deficiencies rarely if ever occur, except in infants who do not have intestinal bacteria that manufacture the vitamin. Main uses are medical: e.g., preparatory to surgery, in expectant mothers or infants at birth to prevent hemorrhagic disease of the newborn, in patients with liver or gallbladder disease.

Your vitamin needs

The above is a pretty melancholy list of misfortunes that can befall you if you don't get enough vitamins. It's not a complete list, either. How in the world are you going to pick and choose foods that are rich in this or that vitamin, in just the right amounts for all the family?

Well, matters are even worse than you think. If you are truly deficient in one vitamin, you're almost sure to be deficient in several others. Vitamins work together, depend on each other. They also work hand in hand with factors that are not vitamins at all. Lack of niacin leads to a vitamin-deficiency disease, pellagra. But pellagra can be prevented by protein foods containing an amino acid, tryptophane, one of the twenty-odd "building blocks" of proteins. Tryptophane is converted into niacin, the anti-pellagra vitamin. So, is pellagra a result of vitamin deficiency or protein deficiency?

A severe deficiency of any single vitamin will sooner or later interfere with other vitamins. Vitamins are great overlappers. They seem to bustle around, doing fragments of each other's work as it pleases them, with no respect for jurisdictional lines. Requirements for certain vitamins increase when we step up our carbohydrate intake; for others, when we eat more protein. Fevers, pregnancy, stresses, possibly increasing age, increase our vitamin needs. Your personal vitamin needs may be different from the other fellow's.

These things would be very upsetting if you had to measure your vitamin intake in micrograms. It's easy for a healthy person to get a beautifully balanced vitamin intake. Daily allowances for average persons have been figured for us by the National Research Council. Don't confuse these recommended daily allowances with the *therapeutic* use of vitamins by doctors—doses, perhaps large doses, of vitamins given to correct known deficiencies.

How to get your vitamins

Neanderthal man ate vitamins all his life and never knew it. Through the ages, man has been an omnivorous creature, eating just about anything (if you don't believe it, go without meals for three days). We should be able to get our vitamins from food, as primitive man did, without bothering our heads about it. Trouble is, civilized foods are a little different, and so are our tastes. So a little knowledge about the vitamin values of common foods will help us to balance our diets.

This is not to say that we should analyze the vitamin values of our diet down to the last milligram. The simple way to get your vitamins, without counting, is to eat a generous *variety* of protective foods. Some foods are rich in certain vitamins, poor in others. Their superiorities and deficiencies tend to strike a balance if we eat omnivorously, as nature seemingly intended.

Very few foods, except fortified milk or some seafoods, furnish vitamin D. This doesn't matter to most adults, whose sunlit skins make all of the vitamin they need. If your food supplies all the vitamins that we have talked about, it's a pretty safe bet that you're getting ample amounts of all the others, including some that still await discovery.

Some foods contain no vitamins at all, or so few that they aren't worth counting. They are excellent, appetite-satisfying foods, important sources of calories in the average diet. But they're so delicious and tempting that we can easily consume excessive amounts of them. If we do, we dilute the vitamin values of our diet.

Don't forget that the *calories* furnished by fats, oils, and sugars are important unless you're trying to lose weight. But you can see why a balanced reducing diet, which in the main is made up of vitamin-rich foods, comes pretty close to supplying as many vitamins as the general diets of people who aren't reducing.

A word about vitamin pills

A vitamin is a vitamin whether it comes from a pill or a cabbage. The vitamins contained in capsules you buy at the drugstore are precisely the same, and do you as much good, as the ones you eat at dinner. Whether an adult in reasonably good health needs vitamin supplements is a question you'd better have your doctor answer. It's especially unwise to decide all by yourself that you need large doses of some single vitamin—say, thiamin for your nerves, or Vitamin A to prevent colds. You might unbalance the teeter-totter. While most vitamins, if taken to excess, are simply excreted with no damage except to your wallet, huge, long-continued doses of vitamins A or D can produce toxic symptoms.

Chapter 15

Cut calories, but
enjoy variety

Don't be too solemn about calorie counting. You don't have to record every calorie as meticulously, and apprehensively, as if it were an item in your income tax report. We'll let you in on a secret: tables can't be accurate down to the last split calorie for all the foods you eat. Nor does this matter in the least. Whether the carrot you eat contains 31 calories, instead of 21, makes no practical difference. So don't chop an inch off a carrot, to make it conform to some standard size listed in a food chart. You don't weigh your food by the gram, as the experts do when they make calorie calculations. You eat average portions (well, maybe double-average), and use common household measuring units. The values in this table are so listed, because that's the way you eat. These measurements are bound to vary slightly; we're only human. But you can believe this: The calorie table is sufficiently, if not offensively, accurate to tell you all you need to know about the food energy that is or isn't getting into you.

Mainly, a calorie table reveals things about food your eyes can't see. The eye is easily deceived by mere size of a food portion. You can gorge on cucumbers all day, yet get hardly enough calories to keep a sparrow alive, but a few tablespoons of a fancy dressing can quickly add up to nearly all the calories allowed in a reducing diet. Other surprising differences in calorie values will show up as you refer to the table, and after a while you will find that you can make a very close estimate of the calories you eat, without studying a chart. Thus you are perpetually protected, as far as knowledge goes, when your hostess offers you a puzzling choice between a super-rich dessert and a strip of celery. Let the calorie table be a friendly guide, not a slide rule to crack over your conscience.

Do make a habit of listing the calories of everything that gets into you via your mouth—drinkables as well as eatables. Keep a pad and pencil handy, add up the score card at the end of the day. Count the nibbles, the tastes you sneak while cooking, the leftover olive you swallow in the interests of tidiness (too good to waste, too insignificant to store in the refrigerator). You may be surprised! This score-card habit helps to keep you from taking that extra roll, or that second helping of truffles, when you visualize the added food as so much extra fat on your frame. In time, you'll recognize such threats on sight and won't have to keep a detailed score. A new learned habit will replace an old upholstering habit.

Remember that calories tell nothing about the *quality* of the foods you eat. Some perfectly good foods provide calories but no vitamins, minerals, or proteins whatever. Don't rule them out of your life on that account. Most of us need reasonable amounts of high-calorie foods, because otherwise we'd have to eat fantastic amounts of low-calorie foods to satisfy our energy needs.

Of course, if we are reducing, our problem is too many calories, and we logically cut down on high-calorie foods. But there are people who find it difficult to gain weight, or who deliberately keep themselves overthin, who need more calories. Whether more or fewer calories is the problem, the table gives you a yardstick to measure the heat-energy of your diet. Foods fall into natural groups— meats, vegetables, etc.—and they are so listed in the table, with brief mention of values, other than calories, generally typical of each group. Foods are also listed alphabetically in Chapter 16.

Meat, poultry, fish

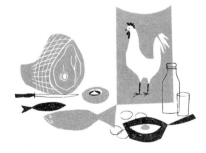

Meat, fish, and poultry contain highest quality protein, and are a good source of minerals. All lean meats are substantially the same in nutritive values, differing mainly in amounts of fat, water, and connective tissue. Organ meats (liver, kidneys, etc.) are higher in vitamins than muscle meats. White and dark poultry meats are nutritionally equal. There is as much protein in white meat as red meat. Fish have the same general value as other forms of meat, and proteins are equally good. Some fish rate relatively high in vitamins A and D; seafoods are good iodine sources.

Editor's note: 1 cup equals 8 fluid ounces and there are 16 tablespoons in 1 cup.

Fish

	Calories
Clams, canned, solids and liquid, 3 ounces	45
Cod, dried, 1 ounce	105
Crabs, Atlantic and Pacific, hard-shell, 3 ounces	90
Flounder, 4 ounces	80
Frog legs, 4 ounces	80
Haddock, fried, 1 fillet	160
Halibut, broiled, 1 steak	230
Herring, smoked, kippered, 3 ounces	180
Lobster, 3 ounces	80
Mackerel, canned, solids and liquid, 3 ounces	155
Salmon:	
Broiled or baked, 1 steak (4x3x½ in.)	205
Canned, solids and liquid (including bones):	
Pink, 3 ounces	120
Sockeye or red, 3 ounces	150
Sardines, canned in oil, drained solids, 3 ounces	180
Scallops, 4 ounces	90
Shad, 4 ounces	190
Shrimp, canned or cooked:	
Wet pack, 3 ounces	75
Swordfish, broiled, 1 steak (3x3x½ in.)	225
Tuna, canned, 3 ounces	170

Fish extras

	Calories
Creole sauce, ¼ cup	100
Drawn butter, 1 tablespoon	110
Lemon wedge, 1 tablespoon	5
Tartare sauce, 1 tablespoon	100

Meat

	Calories
Bacon, medium fat, broiled or fried, 2 slices	95
Bacon, Canadian, 1 slice	65
Beef, canned:	
Corned beef, medium fat, 3 ounces	180
Corned-beef hash, 3 ounces	120
Roast beef, 3 ounces	190
Beef cuts, cooked:	
Chuck, 3 ounces without bone	265
Hamburger, 3 ounces	315
Porterhouse, 3 ounces without bone	295
Rib roast, 3 ounces without bone	265
Round, 3 ounces without bone	195
Rump, 3 ounces without bone	320
Sirloin, 3 ounces without bone	255

Beef, dried or chipped,
2 ounces................115
Beef-and-vegetable stew,
1 cup..................250
Brains, all kinds, 3 ounces....105
Chicken:
Broiled, ½ bird (8 ounces,
bone out)..............330
Canned, boned, 3 ounces...170
Fried, 1 thigh and 1 leg....330
Hens, stewing chickens
(4 ounces).............340
Roasted (4 ounces,
bone out)..............225
Salad, with lettuce, ½ cup.150
Duck, roast, ¼ breast and
1 thigh.................170
Heart, beef, 3 ounces.........90
Kidneys:
Beef, 3 ounces...........120
Lamb, 3 ounces..........90
Pork, 3 ounces............95
Lamb:
Leg roast, 3 ounces
without bone..........230
Rib chop, 3 ounces
without bone..........355
Shoulder roast, 3 ounces
without bone..........295
Liver, beef, 3 ounces........120
Pork:
Cured:
Ham, smoked, cooked:
3 ounces without bone.340
Fresh, cooked:
Ham, 3 ounces
without bone.........340
Loin or chops:
1 chop.............295
3 ounces without bone.285
Spareribs, 4 ribs........330
Luncheon meat:
Boiled ham, 2 ounces....170
Canned, spiced, 2 ounces.165
Sausage:
Bologna, 1 piece (1x1½ in.).465
Frankfurter, 1 frankfurter..125
Liver, liverwurst, 2 ounces..150
Pork, bulk, 4 ounces or
cooked................340

Vienna sausage, 4 ounces...245
Spaghetti with meat sauce,
1 cup..................290
Spanish rice, ¾ cup........155
Tongue, beef, 4 ounces......235
Turkey, medium fat, 4 ounces.305
Veal, cooked:
Cutlet, 3 ounces
without bone..........185
Shoulder roast, 3 ounces
without bone..........195
Stew meat, 3 ounces
without bone..........250

Meat extras

Bread stuffing, ½ cup.......170
Catsup, 1 tablespoon........ 15
Chili sauce, 1 tablespoon..... 15
Gravy, ¼ cup...............75
Tomato puree, ¼ cup........20

Soups

                              Calories
Bouillon cubes, 1 cube.........2
Oyster stew, 1 cup
(with 3-4 oysters)........210
Soups, canned:
Bean, ready-to-serve, 1 cup.190
Beef, ready-to-serve, 1 cup..100
Bouillon, broth, and
consommé, ready-to-
serve, 1 cup............10
Chicken, ready-to-serve,
1 cup..................75
Clam chowder, ready-to-
serve, 1 cup............85
Cream soup (asparagus,
or mushroom) ready-to-
serve, 1 cup...........200
Noodle, rice, or barley,
ready-to-serve, 1 cup....115
Onion, ready-to-serve,
1 cup..................60
Pea, ready-to-serve, 1 cup..140
Tomato, ready-to-serve,
1 cup..................90
Vegetable, ready-to-serve,
1 cup..................80

Eggs

Eggs contain highest quality protein. Practically all the vitamins and most of the fat are in the yolk. The yolk has excellent vitamin values, except vitamin C.

Eggs

Calories

Eggs:
Cooked in shell, 1 egg..... 75
Fried, 1 egg..............105

Omelet, 1-egg omelet......105
Poached, 1 medium egg.... 75
Scrambled, 1 egg.........105

Milk, cheese, cream

Milk protein is of very highest quality. Milk contains all necessary vitamins and minerals, but not all in ideal amounts (low in iron, vitamin C). It is rich in calcium, which is next to impossible to obtain in adequate amounts from other dietary sources. Skim milk, including buttermilk, has practically the same nutritional values as an equal amount of whole milk, except for fewer calories and loss of fat-soluble vitamins (especially vitamin A). Cheese made from whole milk, such as Cheddar or American, can in general be substituted for whole milk at rate of $1\frac{1}{2}$ ounces of cheese for 1 cup of fluid milk.

Milk

Calories

Buttermilk, cultured
(from skim milk), 1 cup.....85
Chocolate beverage
(made with milk), 1 cup...240
Cocoa beverage

(made with milk), 1 cup...235
Milk:
Malted, 1 cup............280
Nonfat (skim), 1 cup......85
Whole, 1 cup.............165

Cheese

Calories
Cheese:
  American or Cheddar,
    1 ounce (1-in. cube).....115
  American or Cheddar
    process, 1 ounce........105
  Blue, 1 ounce............105
  Camembert, 1 ounce.......85

Cheese foods, 1 ounce......90
Cottage, from skim milk,
  1 cup.................215
Cream cheese, 1 ounce.....105
Limburger, 1 ounce.......95
Parmesan, 1 ounce........110
Swiss, 1 ounce............105
Swiss, process, 1 ounce.....100

Macaroni and cheese, 1 cup..465

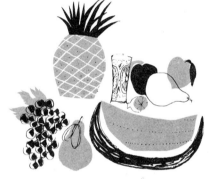

Fruits and juices

    Fruits and juices are especially valued for vitamins, appetizing flavor, laxative properties. Most of the calories come from natural sugars that are quickly utilized. There is considerable variation in vitamin content among different fruits.

Fruits and juices

Calories
Apples, 1 medium...........75
Applesauce, 1 cup sweetened.185
Applesauce, 1cup unsweetened 100
Apricots:
  Dried, cooked, unsweetened,
    fruit and liquid, 1 cup
    (approx. 25 halves)......240

Raw, 3 apricots............55
Syrup pack, 4 medium
  halves and 2 tablespoons
  syrup................95
Avocado, ½ peeled
  (3½x3¼ in.)............280
Bananas, 1 medium (6x1½ in.).90
Blackberries:
  Canned, solids and liquid,
    syrup pack, 1 cup.......215

Raw, 1 cup. 80

Blueberries:
Frozen, without sugar,
3 ounces. 50
Raw, 1 cup. 85
Syrup pack, 1 cup. 245

Cantaloupe, ½ melon
(5 in. diam.). 35

Cherries, 1 cup, pitted. 95

Cranberry sauce, ¼ cup. 135

Figs, canned, syrup pack,
3 figs and 2 tablespoons
syrup. 130

Fruit cocktail, 1 cup. 180

Grapefruit:
Canned in syrup, solids and
liquid, 1 cup. 180
Raw, ½ medium
(4¼ in. diam.). 75

Grapes, raw:
Concord, 1 cup with
skins and seeds. 85
Tokay, Thompson seedless,
1 cup. 100

Honeydew melon, 1 wedge
(2x7 in.). 50

Oranges, 1 medium
(3 in. diam.). 70

Peaches:
Canned, syrup pack, 2
medium-size halves plus
2 tablespoons syrup. 80
Dried, cooked, no sugar
added, 1 cup. 225
Frozen, 4 ounces. 90
Raw, 1 medium. 45

Pears:
Canned, syrup pack,
2 medium-size halves. . . . 80
Raw, 1 pear. 95

Pineapple:
Canned, syurp pack, 2 small
or 1 large slice plus 2
tablespoons juice. 95

Frozen, 4 ounces. 95
Raw, 1 slice (¾ in. thick,
3½ in. diam.). 45

Plums (all, excluding prunes)
raw, 1 plum (2 in. diam.). . .30

Plums (Italian prunes),
canned, 3 prunes (without
pits) plus 2 tablespoons
juice. 90

Prunes, dried:
Cooked, no sugar added,
1 cup, 16-18 prunes
(medium size) and ⅓
cup liquid. 310
Uncooked, 4 medium
prunes, (1½x1x½ in.). . . .75

Raisins, dried, 1 tablespoon. . . .25

Raspberries:
Black, raw, 1 cup. 100
Red, raw, 1 cup. 70
Frozen, 3 ounces. 85

Rhubarb, cooked, sugar
added, 1 cup. 385

Strawberries:
Frozen, 3 ounces. 90
Raw, 1 cup. 55

Tangerines, 1 medium
(2½ in. diam.). 35

Watermelons, wedge,
(4x8 in.). 120

Apple juice, fresh or canned,
1 cup. 125

Grape juice, 1 cup. 170

Grapefruit juice, canned,
sweetened, 1 cup. 130

Grapefruit-orange juice blend,
canned, sweetened, 1 cup. .130

Orange juice, fresh, frozen
concentrate (ready-to-drink),
or canned, 1 cup. 110

Pineapple juice, canned, 1 cup.120

Prune juice, canned, 1 cup. . .170

Tomato juice, 1 cup. 50

Vegetables

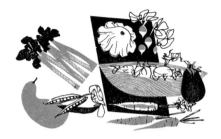

Green leafy vegetables are poor energy sources (low-calorie) but very important for vitamins, minerals, and satisfying bulk. Root vegetables, especially potatoes, are low-cost energy foods (carbohydrate). And are good sources of vitamins and minerals. Yellow vegetables have excellent vitamin A values. Some vegetable minerals and vitamins are dissolved in cooking water; use "pot likker" in soups, gravies. Vegetables counteract acid-forming tendencies of meats and cereals. Vegetables contribute protein which, though usually incomplete, is a valuable part of the average diet, especially if supplemented by such complete proteins as are found in milk products, eggs, and meats.

Vegetables

	Calories
Asparagus, 1 cup cut spears	35
Beans:	
Baby lima, 1 cup	150
Canned, baked, pork and tomato sauce, 1 cup	295
Green, 1 cup	25
Red kidney, canned (or cooked), solids and liquid, 1 cup	230
Wax or yellow, 1 cup	25
Beet greens, 1 cup	40
Beets, 1 cup diced	70
Broccoli, 1 cup	45
Brussels sprouts, 1 cup	60
Cabbage:	
Cooked, 1 cup	40
Raw, 1 cup (shredded finely)	25
Carrots:	
Cooked, 1 cup diced	45
Raw, 1 carrot (5½x1 in.)	20
Cauliflower, cooked, 1 cup	30
Celery, bleached:	

Raw, 1 large outer stalk (8
in. long) 7
Cooked, 1 cup diced 25
Chard, 1 cup 45
Corn, sweet:
1 cup 140
1 ear (5 in. long, 1¾ in.
diam.) 85
Kale, cooked, 1 cup 45
Lettuce:
1 head, compact 70
1 head, loose-leaf 30
2 large or 4 small leaves 7
Mushrooms, canned, solids
and liquid, 1 cup 30
Mustard greens, cooked, 1 cup . 30
Okra, 8 pods (3 in. long,
⅝ in. diam.) 30
Onions:
Cooked, whole, 1 cup 80
Raw, 1 onion (2½ in.
diam.) 50
Young green, 6 small
without tops 25
Parsnips, 1 cup 95
Peas, 1 cup 110
Peppers, green, 1 medium 15
Potatoes:
Baked, 1 medium potato
(2½ in. diam.) 95
Boiled, steamed or pressure-
cooked, 1 medium potato
(2½ in. diam.) or
1 cup diced 105
French-fried, 8 pieces
(2x½x½ in.) 155
Fried raw, 1 cup 480
Hash-browned, 1 cup 470
Mashed, milk added, no
butter, 1 cup 160
Radishes, raw, 4 small 5
Rutabagas, 1 cup cubed or
sliced 50
Sauerkraut, canned, drained,
1 cup 40
Spinach, cooked, 1 cup 45
Squash, summer, 1 cup 35
Squash, winter, baked, 1 cup . . 95
Sweet potatoes, cooked:

Baked, 1 sweet potato
(5x2 in.) 185
Boiled, 1 sweet potato,
(5x2½ in.) 250
Candied, 1 small sweet
potato (3½x2¼ in.) 315
Tomatoes:
Canned or cooked, 1 cup 45
Raw, 1 medium (2x2½ in.) . . 30
Turnips, 1 cup 45

Vegetable extras

Butter or margarine,
1 tablespoon 100
Hollandaise sauce 50
White sauce, medium, ¼ cup . 110

Salads

                                    Calories
Aspic, ½ cup 30
Chef's salad bowl, 1 serving . . 205
Coleslaw, ½ cup, with
mayonnaise 55
Perfection salad, ½ cup 35
Potato salad, ½ cup 200
Waldorf salad, ½ cup 240

Salad extras

Blue-cheese dressing,
Commercial salad dressing, 1
tablespoon 60
Cooked homemade salad
dressing, 1 tablespoon 30
French dressing, 1 tablespoon . . 60
Mayonnaise, 1 tablespoon 90
Olives, mammoth size, 1 olive:
Green 7
Ripe 10
Pickles:
Dill, 1 large 15
Sliced cucumber, 6 slices 30
Sweet cucumber, 1 pickle . . . 20
Russian dressing,
2 tablespoons 150
Salad oil, 1 tablespoon 125
Vinegar, 1 tablespoon 5

Dried beans and peas; nuts

In the dried state, beans and peas, pound for pound, contain more protein than meat—though perhaps not as good as meat protein. Cereals, beans, and peas supplement each other's proteins most valuably. Most nuts contain good protein and considerable fat which steps up calorie value. Beans, peas, and nuts are generally good sources of B vitamins and of some minerals.

Fats and oils

Fats are the most concentrated source of calories (more than twice as many calories as same amounts of protein or carbohydrate). They have "staying power" because they are slow to leave the stomach. In general, fats and oils contain no vitamins, minerals, or proteins, except butter, cream, and margarine which are excellent sources of vitamin A.

Cereals, flours, breads

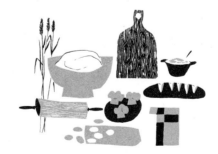

Cereals are rich in carbohydrates, and are important as cheap energy sources. Whole grains are valuable vitamin and mineral sources. Many values, lost in milling, are restored by "enrichment." Enriched white flour contains more iron, thiamin, riboflavin, and niacin than unenriched flour. Cereal and vegetable proteins are incomplete (lack or are deficient in one or more essential amino acids), but one tends to make up for protein deficiencies of another, if eaten together. Value of cereal protein is enhanced if supplemented with milk or other complete-protein foods. Added milk solids increase protein values of breads and baked goods. Cereals and breads in themselves are not excessively high in calories, considering the values they contribute to the diet.

Breads and grain

Calories

Biscuits, baking powder,
1 biscuit (2½ in. diam.)...130
Bran (breakfast cereal), 1 cup.145
Bran flakes (40 percent bran),
1 cup....................115
Bran muffins, 2 small........100
Bran, raisin, 1 cup..........150
Breads:
Boston brown bread,
1 slice (3x¾ in.).........105
Cracked-wheat bread,
1 slice(½ in. thick).......60
Raisin bread, 1 slice (½ in.
thick)...................65
Rye bread, American, 1
slice (½ in. thick)........55
White bread:
1 slice (½ in. thick).......65
Toasted, 1 slice...........65
Whole-wheat bread,
1 slice (½ in. thick).....55
Breakfast foods, mixed cereals:
Corn-and-soy grits,
ready-to-eat, 1 cup......175
Grape-Nuts, 1 cup.........410

Corn bread or muffins,
1 muffin (2¾ in. diam.)...105
Corn flakes, 1 cup..........95
Corn meal, yellow or white,
cooked, 1 cup............120
Crackers:
Graham, 2 medium squares.55
Saltines, 2 crackers........35
Soda, plain:
2 crackers (2½ in square).45
10 oyster crackers or 1
tablespoon cracker meal..45
Farina, 1 cup, cooked........105
Macaroni, cooked, 1 cup.....210
Melba toast, 1 slice..........25
Muffins, 1 muffin
(2¾ in. diam.)...........135
Noodles, cooked, 1 cup......105
Oat cereal, ready-to-eat, 1 cup.100
Rice, white, cooked, 1 cup...200
Rice cereals:
Flakes, 1 cup..............120
Puffed, 1 cup...............55
Oatmeal, cooked, 1 cup......150
Rolls:
Plain, 1 roll...............120
Sweet, 1 roll...............180
Vienna, 1 roll.............145

Rye wafers (crisp), 2 wafers
(1⅞x3½ in.) 45
Shortbread (2 squares,
1¾x1¾ in.) 80
Spaghetti, cooked, 1 cup 220
Wheat cereals:
 Flakes, 1 cup 125
 Germ, 1 tablespoon 15
 Puffed, 1 cup 45
 Shredded:
  Plain:
   1 large biscuit
    (4x2¼ in.) 100
   1 round biscuit 85
  With added malt
   and sugar:
   1 cup bite-size biscuits . 215

Extras with bread

Apple butter, 1 tablespoon 35
Butter, 1 pat or square 50

Honey, 1 tablespoon 60
Jams, marmalades, preserves,
 1 tablespoon 55
Jelly, 1 tablespoon 50
Maple syrup, 1 tablespoon 50
Margarine, 1 pat or square 50
Molasses, 1 tablespoon 50
Peanut butter, 1 tablespoon . . . 90
Syrup, table blends (chiefly
 corn syrup), 1 tablespoon . . . 55

Sandwiches

	Calories
Bacon and tomato, 2 slices bread	290
Corned beef, 2 slices bread	345
Cheese, 2 slices bread	325
Ham, 2 slices bread	300
Hamburger, 1 bun	390
Peanut butter, 2 slices bread	365

Sugars and sweets

Sugar is concentrated carbohydrate, easily digested, and quickly utilized. It has high appetite-satisfying value, hence the general custom of a sweet dessert to top off a meal. Refined sugars are devoid of vitamins and minerals, but many protective foods contain forms of sugar (e.g., lactose of milk) along with other nutritive elements.

Desserts

	Calories
Apple betty, 1 cup	345
Blancmange (vanilla corn-starch pudding), 1 cup	275
Cakes, unfrosted:	
Angel (1/16 of a 10-in. cake)	105

	Calories
Chocolate (1/16 of a 8-in. cake)	200
Lemon chiffon (2x2-in. piece)	105
Spice cake (1/16 of a 9-in. cake)	240
White cake (1/16 of a 9-in. cake)	230

Yellow cake (1/16 of a
9-in. cake)............125
Cheese cake (3-in. wedge)....300
Cookies, 2 wafers
(2⅛ in. diam.)............45
Cream puff, 1 small........150
Custard, baked, ½ cup......140
Doughnut, cake-type, 1......135
Fig bars, 1 large............85
Gelatin dessert, ready-to-serve,
plain, 1 cup............155
Gingerbread, 1 piece
(2x2x2 in.)..............180
Ice, lemon or orange, ½ cup..155
Ice cream:
Chocolate, ½ cup........200
Vanilla, ½ cup..........160
Pies:
Apple (⅙ of a 9-in pie)....505
Blueberry (⅙ of an
8-in. pie).............460
Cherry (⅙ of a 9-in. pie)..510
Custard (⅙ of a 9-in. pie)..275
Lemon meringue (⅙ of a
9-in. pie).............475
Pumpkin (1/6 of a 9-in. pie) 340
Prune whip, 1 cup.........200
Sherbet, ½ cup............120
Strawberry shortcake (old-
fashioned biscuit), with
whipped cream..........300

Dessert extras

Chocolate syrup, 1 tablespoon..40
Chopped peanuts,
1 tablespoon..............50
Hard sauce, 1 tablespoon.....100
Whipped cream, 1 tablespoon..35

Temptations

Calories

Candy:
Butterscotch, 1 ounce......115
Caramels, 1 ounce........120
Chocolate, sweetened,
milk, 1 ounce..........145
Chocolate, sweetened, milk,
with almonds, 1 ounce...150
Chocolate creams, 1 ounce.110
Fondant, 1 ounce........100
Fudge, plain, 1 ounce.....115
Gumdrops, 5 small........25
Hard, 1 ounce...........110
Marshmallow, 1 ounce......90
Mint, (1 in. diam.).........35
Peanut brittle, 1 ounce.....125
Malted milk, all flavors,
10 ounces...............450
Nuts:
Almonds, salted, 10 to 12...100
Brazil, 1.................45
Cashew, 1................20
Filberts, 6...............50
Peanuts, 10 kernels........55
Pecan, 1 half.............10
Walnut, 1 half............10
Popcorn, popped, 1 cup.......55
Potato chips, 7 large........110
Pretzels, 5 small sticks........20
Sodas, ice cream, all flavors...350
Sundaes:
Chocolate ice cream,
chocolate sauce,
nut-sprinkled..........425
Fruit ice cream, fruit sauce.250
Vanilla, marshmallow
sauce, nut-sprinkled.....350

Chapter 16

Your
calorie list
from A to Z

This list is alphabetized for easy counting. Remember: 16 tablespoons or 8 fluid ounces equal one measuring cup, and you can tailor the figures to fit what you eat. Don't cheat by measuring with teacups and serving spoons!

a
Calories

Almonds:
  1 cup. 850
  10–12 salted. 100

Apples:
  1 cup cubed or sliced. 85
  1 medium (2½ in. diam.). . . .75

Apple betty, 1 cup. 345

Apple butter, 1 tablespoon. . . .35

Apple juice, fresh or canned,
  1 cup. 125

Applesauce:
  Sweetened, 1 cup. 185
  Unsweetened, 1 cup. 100

Apricots:
  Canned
    Syrup pack
      1 cup halves and syrup. 205
      4 medium halves and
        2 tablespoons syrup. . 95
    Water pack, 1 cup halves
      and liquid. 75
  Dried
    Cooked, sweetened, fruit
      and syrup
      1 cup (approx. 25
        halves). 400
    Cooked, unsweetened,

fruit and liquid
1 cup (approx. 25
halves)..........240
Frozen, 3 ounces...........70
Raw, 3 apricots............55
Asparagus, 1 cup cut spears...35
Avocados:
1 cup (½-in. cubes)......370
½ peeled avocado
(3½x3¼ in.)...........280

b

Bacon, Canadian, 1 slice......65
Bacon, medium fat, broiled
or fried, 2 slices............95
Bacon-and-tomato sandwich, 2
slices bread, 2 slices bacon,
½ tomato, 1 pat butter....290
Bananas:
1 cup slices..............135
1 medium (6x1½ in.)......90
Beans:
Baby lima, 1 cup.........150
Canned, baked
Pork and molasses, 1 cup.325
Pork and tomato sauce,
1 cup................295
Green, 1 cup..............25
Red kidney
Canned (or cooked), sol-
ids and liquid, 1 cup..230
Wax or yellow, 1 cup.......25
Beef cuts, cooked:
Chuck (pot roast)
3 ounces without bone...265
1 pound with bone....1,140
Hamburger
3 ounces..............315
1 pound.............1,655
Hamburger sandwich, open
face...................390
Rib roast
3 ounces without bone...265
1 pound with bone....1,050

Round
3 ounces without bone...195
1 pound with bone......915
Swiss steak
(3x2½x1½ in.)......320
Rump
3 ounces without bone..320
1 pound with bone....1,170
Steak
3 ounces without bone...270
1 pound with bone....1,400
Beef, canned:
Corned beef, 3 ounces.....180
Corned-beef hash, 3 ounces.120
Beef, dried or chipped:
1 cup...................335
2 ounces................115
Beer (4 percent alcohol),
12 ounces...............170
Beer, bock, 7-ounce glass.....135
Beer (3.2 percent alcohol),
7-ounce glass.............80
Beet greens, 1 cup..........40
Beets, 1 cup diced..........70
Benedictine, ⅔-ounce glass....75
Beverages, carbonated:
Ginger ale, 8 fluid ounces...80
Other, including cola type,
6 fluid ounces..........85
Biscuits, baking powder, 1
biscuit (2½ in. diam.).....130
Bitters, 1 dash..............10
Blackberries:
Canned, solids and liquid
Syrup pack, 1 cup.....215
Water pack, 1 cup......105
Raw, 1 cup..............80
Blancmange (vanilla corn-
starch pudding), 1 cup....275
Blueberries:
Canned, solids and liquid
Syrup pack, 1 cup......245
Water pack, 1 cup.......90
Frozen, without sugar,
3 ounces...............50
Raw, 1 cup..............85

Blue-cheese dressing, 2
tablespoons.............150

Bouillon cube.................2

Bourbon, 1½-ounce jigger...130

Brains, all kinds, 3 ounces....105

Bran (breakfast cereal) 1 cup.145

Bran flakes (40 percent
bran), 1 cup.............115

Bran muffins, 2 small.......100

Bran, raisin, 1 cup.........150

Brazil nuts:
Shelled, 1 cup...........905
1 Brazil nut..............45

Bread crumbs, dry, 1 cup....340

Breads:
Boston brown bread, 1
slice (3x¾ in.)..........105
Raisin bread, 1 slice (½
in. thick)..............65
Rye bread, American, 1
slice (½ in. thick).......55
White bread:
1 slice (½ in. thick).....65
1 slice, toasted..........65
Whole-wheat bread, 1
slice (½ in. thick).......55

Breakfast foods, mixed
cereals, wheat and malted
barley, 1 cup..........410

Broccoli, 1 cup.............45

Brussels sprouts, 1 cup.......60

Burgundy, 3-ounce glass.......75

Butter:
1 cup..................1,605
1 pat or square..........50
1 tablespoon.............100

Buttermilk, cultured (made
from skim milk), 1 cup.....85

C

Cabbage:
Cooked, 1 cup............40
Raw, 1 cup, finely
shredded...............25

Cakes:
Angel (1/16 of a
10-in. cake)...........105
Butter sponge (1/16 of a
9-in. cake)............180
Chocolate (1/16 of an
8-in. cake)............200
Lemon chiffon
(piece 2x2-in.).........105
Spice (1/16 of a
9-in. cake)............240
White (1/16 of a
9-in. cake)............230
Yellow (1/16 of a
9-in. cake)............125

Candy:
Butterscotch, 1 ounce......115
Candied or glace peel
Citron, 1 ounce.........90
Ginger root, crystal-
lized, 1 ounce........95
Lemon, orange, or
grapefruit peel, 1 ounce.90
Caramels, 1 ounce.........120
Chocolate, sweetened,
milk, 1 ounce..........145
Chocolate, sweetened,
milk, with almonds,
1 ounce..............150
Chocolate creams, 1 ounce.110
Fondant, 1 ounce.........100
Fudge, plain, 1 ounce.....115
Gumdrops, 5 small.........25
Hard, 1 ounce............110
Marshallows, 1 ounce.......90
Mint, 1, 1 in. diameter.....35
Peanut brittle, 1 ounce....125

Cantaloupes:
½ melon (5 in. diam.)......35
1 cup diced...............30

Carrots:
Cooked, 1 cup diced.......45
Raw
1 carrot (5½x1 in.)......20
1 cup grated............45

Cashew nuts:
  1 cashew nut..............20
  1 ounce.................165
Catawba, 3-ounce glass......140
Cauliflower:
  Cooked, 1 cup............30
  Raw, 1 cup cauliflowerets...25
Celery, bleached:
  Cooked, 1 cup diced.......25
  Raw
    1 cup diced.............20
    1 large outer stalk
      (8 in. long)............5
Champagne:
  Dry, 3-ounce glass.........90
  Sweet, 3-ounce glass......120
Chard leaves, 1 cup cooked...45
Chartreuse, ⅔-ounce glass.....75
Cheese:
  American or Cheddar
    1 cup, grated..........445
    1 ounce (1-in. cube).....115
  American or Cheddar,
    process, 1 ounce........105
  Blue, 1 ounce............105
  Camembert, 1 ounce......85
  Cheese foods, 1 ounce.....90
  Cottage, from skim milk,
    1 cup.................215
  Cream cheese
    1 ounce...............105
    1 tablespoon............55
  Limburger, 1 ounce........95
  Parmesan, 1 ounce.......110
  Swiss, 1 ounce...........105
  Swiss, process, 1 ounce.....100
Cheese cake, 3-in. wedge.....300
Cheese sandwich...........325
Chef's salad bowl...........85
Cherries, 1 cup, pitted.......95
Cherries, red, sour, pitted,
  canned, 1 cup...........120
Chianti, 3-ounce glass........75
Chicken:
  Broilers, ½ bird (8 ounces,
    bone out).............330

Canned, boned, 3 ounces...170
Creamed, ½ cup........160
Fried, thigh, 1 leg.......330
Hens, stewing chickens
  (4 ounces).............340
Roasters (4 ounces, bone
  out)..................225
Salad, with lettuce, ½ cup..150
Chili sauce, 1 tablespoon......15
Chocolate:
  Sweetened, plain, 1 square..135
  Unsweetened, 1 square.....140
Chocolate beverage, made
  with milk, 1 cup.........240
Chocolate syrup, 1
  tablespoon...............40
Clams:
  Canned, solids and liquid,
    3 ounces...............45
  Raw, 4 ounces............90
Claret, 3-ounce glass.........75
Cocoa beverage, made with
  all milk, 1 cup...........235
Cocoa, breakfast, plain, dry
  powder:
    1 cup, stirred before
      measuring...........330
    1 tablespoon...........20
Coconut:
  Dried, 1 cup.............345
  Fresh, 1 cup shredded.....350
Cod:
  Dried, 1 ounce...........105
  Raw, 4 ounces............85
Coffee......................0
Cointreau, ⅔-ounce glass......75
Coleslaw, 1 cup............100
Cookies, plain and assorted:
  1 cooky (3 in. diam., ½ in.
    thick).................110
  2 wafers (2⅛ in. diam.).....45
Corn, sweet:
  1 cup..................140
  1 ear (5 in. long, 1¾ in.
    diam.).................85

Corn bread or muffins, 1
muffin (2¾ in. diam.).....105

Corn flakes, 1 cup..........95

Corn meal, yellow or white
Cooked, 1 cup...........120
Dry, 1 cup.............525

Cornstarch, 1 tablespoon......30

Corn syrup, 1 tablespoon.....55

Crabs, Atlantic and Pacific,
hard-shell, 3 ounces........90

Crackers:
Graham, 4 small or
2 medium squares.......55
Saltines, 2 crackers (2-in.
square)...............35
Soda, plain
2 crackers (2½-in.
square)..............45
10 oyster crackers or 1
tablespoon cracker meal. 45

Cream puff, 1 small........150

Creme de menthe, ⅔-ounce
glass....................75

Creme de cacao, ⅔-ounce
glass....................75

Creole sauce, ¼ cup........100

Curacao, ⅔-ounce glass.......75

Custard, baked, ½ cup......140

d

Dates, "fresh" and dried,
1 cup, pitted.............505

Doughnut, cake type, 1......135

Drawn butter, 1 tablespoon..110

Duck, roast, ¼ breast and
1 thigh.................170

e

Eggs:
Omelet, 1-egg omelet......105
Scrambled, 1 egg.........105
White, 1 egg white........15
Whole, cooked in shell or
poached...............75
Yolk, 1 egg yolk...........60

Endive or escarole, 1 pound...90

f

Farina, 1 cup cooked.......105

Fats, cooking (vegetable):
1 cup.................1,770
1 tablespoon............110

Figs:
Canned, syrup pack, 3 figs
and 2 tablespoons syrup. 130
Dried, 1 large (2x1 in.).....55

Fig bars, 1 large............85

Filbert nuts, 6..............50

Flounder, 4 ounces..........80

Frog legs, 4 ounces..........80

Fruit cocktail, 1 cup.........180

g

Gelatin, dry:
Dessert powder,
3-ounce package.......325
Plain, 1 tablespoon........35

Gelatin dessert, ready-to-
serve, plain, 1 cup........155

Gin, 1½-ounce jigger........130

Gingerbread, 1 piece
(2x2x2 in.)...............180

Grapefruit:
Canned in syrup, solids
and liquid, 1 cup.......180
Raw
½ medium (4¼ in. diam.) 75
1 cup sections...........75

Grapefruit juice:
Canned
Sweetened, 1 cup.......130
Unsweetened, 1 cup......90
Concentrate, frozen,
1 6-ounce can..........295

Grapefruit-orange juice blend:
Canned
Sweetened, 1 cup.......130
Unsweetened, 1 cup.....100
Frozen concentrate,
1 6-ounce can..........295

Grape juice, 1 cup..........170

Grapes, raw:
Concord, 1 cup with
skins and seeds...........85
Tokay, Thompson
seedless, 1 cup..........100

Gravy, ¼ cup...............75

Grenadine, 1 ounce..........75

h

Haddock, cooked, fried:
1 fillet...................160
1 pound.................675

Halibut, broiled:
1 pound.................825
1 steak (4x3x½ in.).......230

Hard sauce, 1 tablespoon....100

Heart, beef, 3 ounces........90

Herring, smoked, kippered,
3 ounces................180

Hollandaise sauce,
1 tablespoon..............50

Honey, 1 tablespoon.........60

Honeydew melon,
1 wedge (2x7 in.).........50

i-j-k

Ice, lemon or orange, ½ cup.155

Ice cream, chocolate, ½ cup.200

Ice cream, vanilla, ½ cup....160

Ice-cream soda, any flavor...350

Jams, marmalades, preserves,
1 tablespoon..............55

Jellies, 1 tablespoon.........50

Kale, cooked, 1 cup.........45

Kidneys:
Beef, 3 ounces............120
Lamb, 3 ounces..........90
Pork, 3 ounces............95

l

Lamb:
Leg roast
3 ounces without bone...230
1 pound.............1,240
Rib chop
3 ounces without bone...355
1 pound.............1,900
Shoulder roast
3 ounces without bone...295
1 pound.............1,550

Lard:
1 cup.................1,985
1 tablespoon............125

Lemon, 1 medium..........20

Lemon or lime juice (fresh,
frozen, or canned), 1 tablespoon....................4
Lettuce:
  1 head, compact..........70
  1 head, loose-leaf..........30
  2 large or 4 small leaves......7
Liver, 3 ounces.............120
Lobster, 3 ounces...........80

m-n

Macaroni:
  Cooked, 1 cup (1-in.
    pieces or elbow type)....210
  Dry, 1 cup, elbow type....465
Mackerel, canned, solids
  and liquid...............155
Madeira, 3-ounce glass.......110
Maple syrup, 1 tablespoon....50
Maraschino, ⅔-ounce glass....75
Margarine:
  1 cup..................1,615
  1 pat....................50
  1 tablespoon.............100
Marmalade, orange,
  1 tablespoon..............55
Melba toast, 1 slice..........25
Milk:
  Canned
    Condensed (sweetened),
      1 cup..............980
    Evaporated
      (unsweetened), 1 cup..345
  Dried
    Nonfat solids (skim)
      1 cup..............435
      1 tablespoon..........30
    Whole
      1 cup..............630
      1 tablespoon.........40
  Fresh
    Chocolate flavored, 1
      cup.................185

Half and half (milk and
  cream), 1 cup.........330
Nonfat (skim), 1 cup......85
Whole, 1 cup.............165
Malted
  Beverage, 1 cup........280
  Dry powder, 1 ounce....115
Molasses:
  1 cup...................825
  1 tablespoon.............50
Muffins, 1 muffin (2¾ in.
  diam.)..................135
Mung bean sprouts, 1 cup.....20
Muscatel, 3-ounce glass.......165
Mushrooms, canned, solids
  and liquid, 1 cup..........30
Mustard greens, cooked, 1 cup.30
Noodles (containing egg):
  Cooked, 1 cup............105
  Dry, 1 cup...............280

o

Oat cereal, ready-to-eat,
  1 cup...................100
Oatmeal:
  Cooked, 1 cup............150
  Dry, 1 cup...............310
Oils, salad or cooking:
  1 cup..................1,945
  1 tablespoon.............125
Okra, 8 pods (3 in. long, ⅝
  in. diam.)................30
Olives, "mammoth" size:
  Green, 10 olives...........70
  Ripe, 10 olives...........105
Onions:
  Cooked, whole, 1 cup......80
  Raw
    1 onion (2½ in. diam.)...50
    1 tablespoon chopped......4

Onions, young green, 6 small
without tops 25

Oranges:
1 cup sections 85
1 medium (3 in. diam.) 70

Orange juice:
Canned
Unsweetened, 1 cup 110
Fresh, 1 cup 110
Concentrate, frozen, 1
6-ounce can 300

Oysters, raw, 1 cup (13-19
medium size) 200

Oyster stew, 1 cup with 3-4
oysters 210

p

Pancake mix:
Buckwheat, 1 cup 430
Wheat, 1 cup 470

Pancakes:
Buckwheat, 1 cake (4 in.
diam.) 45
Wheat, 1 cake (4 in. diam.) . . 60

Parsley, 1 tablespoon chopped . . 1

Parsnips, 1 cup 95

Peaches:
Canned, solids and liquid
Syrup pack
1 cup 175
2 medium halves and
2 tablespoons syrup . . . 80
Water pack, 1 cup 65
Dried
Cooked, no sugar added,
1 cup 225
Cooked, sugar added,
1 cup 365
Frozen, 4 ounces 90
Raw
1 cup, sliced 75
1 medium 45

Peanut butter, 1 tablespoon . . . 90

Peanut-butter sandwich 365

Peanuts, shelled:
1 cup medium halves 805
10 kernels 55
1 tablespoon, chopped 50

Pears:
Canned, solids and liquid
Syrup pack
1 cup 175
2 medium-size halves
plus 2 tablespoons
syrup 80
Water pack, 1 cup 75
Raw, 1 pear 95

Peas:
Canned, 1 cup 145
Cooked, 1 cup 110

Pecans:
1 cup, halves 750
1 half 10
1 tablespoon, chopped 50

Peppers, green, 1 medium 15

Perfection salad, ½ cup 35

Pickles:
Dill, 1 large 15
Sliced cucumbers, 6 slices . . . 30
Sweet, cucumber, 1 pickle . . 20

Piecrust, plain:
1 double crust
(for 9-inch pie) 1,485
1 lower crust
(9-in. shell) 740

Pies:
Apple (1/6 of a
9-in. pie) 505
Blueberry (1/6 of an
8-in. pie) 460
Cherry (1/6 of a
9-in. pie) 510
Custard (1/6 of a
9-in. pie) 275
Lemon meringue (1/6 of a
9-in. pie) 475
Pumpkin (1/6 of a
9-in. pie) 340

Pimientos, canned, 1 medium . . 10

Pineapple:
Canned, syrup pack,
solids and liquid
1 cup crushed........205
2 small or 1 large slice
plus 2 tablespoons
juice...........95
Frozen, 4 ounces..........95
Raw
1 cup, diced.............75
1 slice (¾ in. thick,
3½ in. diam.).........45

Pineapple juice, canned,
1 cup..................120

Plums (all, excluding
prunes), raw, 1 plum
(2-in. diam.)............30

Plums (Italian prunes),
canned, syrup pack, 3
prunes (without pits) plus
2 tablespoons juice.....90

Popcorn, popped, 1 cup.......55

Pork:
Cured
Ham, smoked, cooked
3 ounces without bone.340
1 pound with bone..1,495
1 pound without
bone...........1,805
Fresh, cooked
Ham
3 ounces without bone.340
1 pound with bone..1,430
Loin or chops
1 chop..............295
3 ounces without bone.285
1 pound with bone..1,150
Spareribs, 4 ribs.......330
Luncheon meat
Boiled ham, 2 ounces....170
Canned, spiced,
2 ounces.............165

Port, 3–ounce glass..........165

Potatoes:
Baked, 1 medium potato
(2½ in. diam.)..........95

Boiled, steamed, or pressure-
cooked, 1 medium potato

(2½ in. diam.) or 1
cup diced..........105
Canned, 3-4 very small....120
French-fried, 8 pieces
(2x½x½ in.)...........155
Fried raw, 1 cup..........480
Hash-browned, 1 cup.....470
Mashed, milk added,
no butter, 1 cup.......160

Potato chips, 10 medium
(2 in. diam.) or 7 large
(3 in. diam.)..........110

Potato salad, ½ cup........200

Pretzels, 5 small sticks.......20

Prunes, dried:
Cooked, no sugar added
(med. size), 1 cup, 16-18
prunes and ⅓ cup
liquid.............310
Cooked, sugar added (med.
size), 1 cup, 16-18 prunes
and ⅓ cup liquid.....485
Uncooked, 4 medium
prunes, 1½x1x½ in......75

Prune juice, canned, 1 cup...170

Prune whip, 1 cup.........200

Pumpkin, canned, 1 cup......75

r

Radishes, raw, 4 small........5

Raisins:
Dried
1 cup.................430
1 tablespoon............25

Raspberries:
Black, raw, 1 cup........100
Red, raw, 1 cup..........70
Frozen, 3 ounces........85

Rhubarb, cooked, sugar
added, 1 cup.............385

Rice, white, cooked, 1 cup...300

Rice cereals:
Flakes, 1 cup. 120
Puffed, 1 cup. 55
Rolls:
Plain, 1 roll. 120
Sweet, 1 roll. 180
Vienna. 145
Rum, 1½-ounce jigger. 130
Rutabagas, 1 cup cubed
or sliced. 50
Rye, 1½-ounce jigger. 130
Rye flour, light, 1 cup,
sifted. 285
Rye wafers (crisp), 2 wafers
(1⅞x3½ in.). 45

S

Salad dressings:
Commercial, plain
1 cup. 900
1 tablespoon. 60
French
1 cup. 945
1 tablespoon. 60
Home-cooked
1 cup. 445
1 tablespoon. 30
Mayonnaise
1 cup. 1,450
1 tablespoon. 90
Russian dressing, 1
tablespoon. 75
Salmon:
Broiled or baked, 1 steak
(4x3x½-in.). 205
Canned, solids and liquid
(including bones)
Pink, 3 ounces. 120
Sockeye or red, 3 ounces. .145
Sardines, canned in oil,
drained solids, 3 ounces. . . .180
Sauerkraut, canned, drained,
1 cup. 30

Sausage:
Bologna, 1 piece (1x1 ½ in.) 465
Frankfurter, 1. 125
Liver, liverwurst, 2 ounces. .150
Pork, bulk, canned, or
cooked, 4 ounces. 340
Vienna sausage, canned,
4 ounces. 245
Sauterne, California, 3-ounce
glass. 90
Scallops, 4 ounces. 90
Scotch, 1½-ounce jigger. 130
Shad, raw, 4 ounces. 190
Sherbet, ½ cup. 120
Sherry, 3-ounce glass. 140
Shortbread (2 squares,
1¾x1¾ in.). , ...80
Shrimp, canned or cooked:
3 ounces, wet pack. 75
Sloe gin, 1 ounce. 110
Soups, canned:
Bean, ready-to-serve, 1 cup.190
Beef, ready-to-serve, 1 cup. .100
Bouillon, broth, and con-
sommé, ready-to-serve,
1 cup. 10
Chicken, ready-to-serve,
1 cup. 75
Clam chowder, ready-to-
serve, 1 cup. 85
Cream soup (asparagus,
celery, or mushroom),
ready-to-serve, 1 cup. .200
Noodle, rice, or barley,
ready-to-serve, 1 cup. . . .115
Onion, ready-to-serve, 1
cup. 60
Pea, ready-to-serve, 1 cup. .140
Tomato, ready-to-serve,
1 cup. 90
Vegetable, ready-to-serve,
1 cup. 80
Spaghetti, cooked, 1 cup. 220
Spinach, cooked, 1 cup. 45
Squash, summer, 1 cup. 35

Squash, winter, cooked:
Baked, mashed, 1 cup......95
Boiled, mashed, 1 cup......85

Strawberries:
Frozen, 3 ounces..........90
Raw, 1 cup..............55

Strawberry shortcake, with
biscuit, whipped cream....300

Stuffing, bread, ½ cup......170

Sugars:
Brown
1 cup, firm-packed......815
1 tablespoon............50
Confectioner's
1 cup.................495
1 tablespoon...........30
Granulated, cane or beet
1 cup.................770
1 piece, lump sugar
(1⅛x⅝x⅛ in.)........25
1 tablespoon...........50
1 teaspoon.............15
Maple, 1 piece
(1¾x1¼x½ in.)........105

Sundaes:
Chocolate ice cream,
chocolate sauce, nuts....425
Fruit ice cream, fruit sauce.250
Vanilla ice cream, marsh-
mallow sauce, nuts......350

Sweet potatoes:
Canned, 1 cup..........235
Cooked
Baked, 1 sweet potato,
(5x2 in.).............185
Boiled, 1 sweet potato,
(5x2½ in.)...........250
Candied, 1 small sweet
potato (3½x2¼ in.)...315

Swordfish, broiled, 1 steak
(3x3x½ in.)..............225

Syrup, simple, 1 ounce........75

Syrup, table blends (chiefly
corn syrup):
1 cup.................940
1 tablespoon...........55

t

Tangerines, 1 medium
(2½ in. diam.)...........35

Tapioca, dry, 1 cup, granulated quick-cooking, stirred 545

Tartare sauce, 1 tablespoon..100

Tea........................0

Tomato aspic, 1 serving......40

Tomato catsup:
1 cup..................270
1 tablespoon.............15

Tomatoes:
Canned or cooked, 1 cup....45
Raw, 1 medium (2x2½ in.).30

Tomato juice, 1 cup.........50

Tomato puree, canned, 1 cup..90

Tongue, beef, 4 ounces......235

Tuna, canned, drained,
3 ounces...............170

Turkey, medium fat, 4 ounces.305

Turnip greens, 1 cup........45

Turnips, 1 cup.............40

V

Veal, cooked:
Cutlet
3 ounces...............185
1 pound...............995
Shoulder roast
3 ounces without bone...195
1 pound with bone......760
Stew meat
3 ounces...............250
1 pound.............1,345

Vermouth:
French, 1 ounce..........35
Italian, 1 ounce..........60

Vinegar, 1 tablespoon 2
Vodka, 1½-ounce jigger 130

W-y

Waffles, 1 waffle
(4½x5⅝x½ in.) 215
Waldorf salad, ½ cup 240
Walnuts, California:
1 cup halves 655
1 half 10
1 tablespoon chopped 50
Watermelons, wedge
(4x8 in.) 120
Wheat flours:
All-purpose or family flour,
1 cup sifted 400
Cake or pastry flour, 1 cup
sifted 365

Whole wheat, 1 cup 400
Wheat cereals:
Flakes, 1 cup 125
Germ, 1 cup 245
Puffed, 1 cup 45
Shredded
Plain
1 large biscuit
(4x2¼ in.) 100
1 round biscuit 85
With added malt and
sugar
1 cup bite-size
biscuits 215
Whole meal, 1 cup 135
Whipped cream, 1 tablespoon . . 35
White sauce, medium, 1 cup . . 430
Wild rice, raw, 1 cup 595
Yeast:
Compressed, baker's,
1 ounce 25
Dried, brewer's,
1 tablespoon 20

Index

A

A, vitamin............215, 226
  deficiency symptoms......215
  lack of in skim milk......228
  source of...............233

Acid-forming foods.........201

Adolescents
  poor nutrition in.........172
  weight problems......170-174

Alcohol..............203-210
  calories in...............205
  calories not stored........204
  depressant...............203

Alkali-forming foods........202

All about vitamins........*211-222*

Calorie list............237-248

Amino acids............77, 78

Amphetamine.............. 50

Appetite drive...........59, 63

Arteries, hardening of........ 69

B

B vitamins...........216, 217
  source of...............233

Baths, hot, steam........... 48

Behnke, Capitan A. R.......... *19*

Beri beri..................217

Better Homes & Gardens
  Meal Plans............*97-146*

Beverages.................101

Body builds.............18-29
  muscle...............22-24
  plump................. 21
  beanpole............... 21

Breads, value in diet........233

Brozek, Josef.............. *19*

Bland diet.................199

Blood sugar............... 62

Brewer's yeast.............160

Bulk diet..............197-199

Bulk producers............162

Buttermilk................158

C

C, vitamin................218

Calcium.............180-182
  in milk.................228

Calisthenics............51-57

Calorie list
  alcohol..............206-210
  alphabetical..........237-248
  food groups..........225-236
  recipes..............142-146

Calories
  explanation of........... 39
  how to figure requirement.85-94
  in recipe, how to compute..141
  recording of..........58, 224
  requirements...........85-96

Carbohydrates............. 73

Cereals, value in diet.......233

Charts
  calories expended........ 87
  daily-diet diary.......... 60
  height and weight, boys.... 34
  height and weight, girls.... 35
  height and weight, men.... 28
  height and weight, women.. 26
  weight watching.........254

Cheese, value in diet........228
Chlorine..................187
Cocktails, calories in.........209
Constitutional factors........ 20
Cooking methods..........100
Cooley, Donald G............. 5
Cordials, calories in.........208
Cortisone.................. 63
Cottage cheese.............158
Cream, value in diet........228
Cut calories, but enjoy variety. 223-236

D

D, vitamin................218
Deficiency symptoms
    vitamin..............215-219
Diabetes.................68, 69
Diet pack foods, advantage of. 156
Diets, reducing
    protein in............... 83
    safe.................... 72
    satisfying..............94-96
    speed of results..........90-94
Diets, special: see Special diets
Dieting family style........163-178
Dining out.............147-154
    cafeteria.................153
    home................147-149
    lunch counter........151-153
    restaurant...........149-151
Dinitrophenol............. 50
Diseases, degenerative....... 69
Liquors, calories in.........207
Don't overlook calories in
    alcohol...............203-210
Do you need to reduce or gain.. 15-36
Dried beans, value in diet....233

Drinks...............203-210
    cocktails...............209
    cordials..................208
    distilled liquors..........207
    liqueurs..................208
    tall drinks...............209
    malt liquors.............208
    mixed drinks............208
    wines....................206
Dried peas, value in diet.....233
Drugs, in weight reduction. .49-51
Dry skim milk.............158
Dublin, Dr. Louis I........... 69

E

E, vitamin................219
Ectomorph.................20
Eggs, value in diet.........228
Elderly people
    calorie needs of..........166
    cooking for..........165-170
    nutrients in diet...........168
    physical ailments affecting
    appetite.................169
Electric-light cabinets........ 48
Energy, heat.............. 39
Endomorph............... 20
Exercise.................51-57
    value of................51-55
Exercises, see Calisthenics

F

Fat
    areas of deposit........30, 31
    gain and loss of........37-64
    See also Obesity; Reducing
Fats...............73, 74, 233
    value in diet..............233

Fish, value in diet..........225
Flavored gelatin............161
Food as fuel............... 39
Foods, proteins in.........79-83
For safe and sure reducing.....*65-74*
Flours, value in diet.....233, 234
Fresh fruits................157
Fresh vegetable juices........159
Fruit juices, value in diet....229
Fruits, value in diet........229

G-H

Gelatin....................161
Glands in weight problems..41-44
Height and weight
  tables...........26-29, 34, 35
  boys.................... 34
  girls................... 35
  men..................... 28
  women.................. 26
Heredity, relationship with
  obesity.................44-47
High blood pressure.......68, 69
High-residue diets.......197-199
How fat comes and goes.......*37-64*
Hunger pangs.........84, 94-96
Hypothalmus, function of..59, 62

I-K-L

*If the doctor puts you on a
  special diet*.............*191-202*
Introduction to good eating.....*11-14*
Iodine............185-187, 226
Iron....................183-185
  source of................234

K, vitamin................219
Keys, Dr. Ancel..........*196, 32*
Kilander, Dr. H. F............ *45*
Liqueurs, calories in........208
Low-cholesterol diets.....195-197
Low-fat diet...........195-197
Low-salt diet..........192-194
Lunch-box meals........105-108

M-N

Maintaining weight......108-112
Make use of special foods....*155-162*
Malt liquors, calories in......208
Marks, H. H................*69*
Massage................... 48
Meal planning..........97-146
Meal plans............113-140
  1,000 calories....114, 115, 121,
    122, 128, 129, 135, 136
  1,250 calories....116, 117, 123,
    124, 130, 131, 137, 138
  1,500 calories....118, 119, 125,
    126, 132, 133, 139, 140
  Fall.................135-140
  Spring...............121-126
  Summer...............128-133
  Winter...............114-119
Meat, value in diet..........225
Mesomorph................ 20
Milk, value in diet.........228
Minerals................179-190
  calcium..............180-182
  chlorine..................187
  cooking..................190
  iodine..............185-187
  iron.................183-185
  phosphorus..............182
  sodium..................187

Mixed drinks, calories in.....208

McCance, Dr. R. A.........*18, 94*

Neutral foods..............202

Niacin.....................216
    source of.................234

Nonfat dry milk solids.......157

Nutrition................14, 36

Nuts, value in diet.........233

O

Obesity
    causes of...............37-39
    control of, see Reducing
    danger of...............68-70
    types of................63, 64

Overeating................. 39
    reasons for..............58-64

Overweight................ 12
    indications of........24, 30-32
    problems: see Obesity

Oxygen, as fuel............. 40

P

Pellagra...................216

Phosphorus...........182, 183

Poultry, value in diet....225, 226

Proteins.....75-84, 226, 228, 234
    complete................79-83
    composition of.........78-79
    explanation of..........75-77
    foods containing........80-83
    hydrolysates.............162
    need for................ 77
    quality of..............79-83
    in reducing diets.......... 83
    in vegetables............231

Psychic factors in overeating.. 63

R

Rate of reducing........... 87

Reducing..........15-36, 65-74
    diet...................72-74
    drugs.................49-51
    exercise...............51-57
    increasing caloric output..47-49
    methods of............47-58
    protein in............... 83
    rate of................97-99
    reasons for.............66-72
    satisfying diet...........94-96
    speed of results.........90-94
    value of...............70-72

Riboflavin.................216
    source of................234

Rickets....................218

S

Salad dressings.........102-104
    dieter's cooked, recipe.....104
    fruit, recipe.............103
    rosy, recipe..............103

Sandwich recipes...........106

Scurvy....................218

Shaw, Bernard.............. *37*

Sheldon, Dr. Wm. H.......... *20*

Sherman, Dr. Henry C........*181*

Skim milk..................158

Sodium....................187

Sodium-restricted diets...192-194

Special diets...........191-202
    acid-forming foods.......200
    alkali-forming foods...201, 202
    bland...................199
    bulk...................197
    low-cholesterol...........195
    neutral foods............202

sodium restricted......192-194
who needs one............191

Special foods...........155-162
brewer's yeast............160
flavored gelatin..........161
fresh fruits..............157
fresh vegetable juices......159
milk products............158
unflavored gelatin........161
wheat germ.............159

Spices....................101

Specific dynamic action...... 84

Spot reducing appliances..... 49

Substitutions..............107

Sugar, blood.............. 62

Sugars, value in diet........235

Sweeteners................102

Sweets, value in diet........235

T-U

Tall drinks, calories in.......209

Thiamin..................209
source of.................234

Thyroid gland............. 50

Ulcer diet.................199

Underweight...........174-178
frequent meals........175-177
glandular trouble........41-44
problems of..........174-178
relaxation...........177, 178

Unflavored gelatin..........161

V

Vegetables, value in diet.....231

Vitamin,
A.........215, 226, 228, 233
B complex...............216

C...................218, 228
D...................218, 226
E......................219
K......................219

Vitamins,
definition of..........212-214
need for..211-212, 214, 219-220
pills......................222
sources..............220-222

W

Water,
weight of..............45-47
retention of............. 92

Weight and height
tables..........24-29, 34, 35
boys...................... 34
girls..................... 35
men..................... 28
women................. 26

Weight-watching chart......254

Weigh, when to............111

What minerals do for you....179-190

What are your calorie needs?....85-96

Wheat germ...............159

When you're away from home-plate..................147-154

Why proteins are important....75-84

Widdowson, E. M............ 94

Wilson, Dr. James R.......... 9

Wines, calories in...........206

Y

Yeast....................160

Yogurt...................159

Your calorie list from A to Z...............237-248

Score your progress . . .

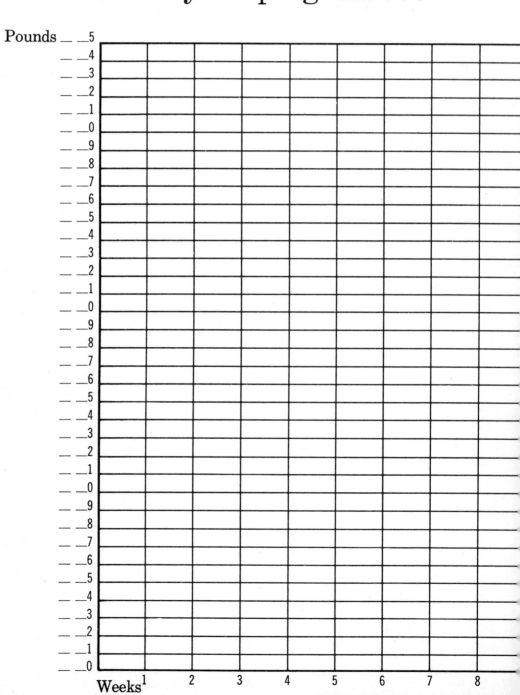

Pounds

This chart is the best check you have on calorie tables. Mark your weight the same time each week. If the line doesn't drop, you're still eating too much. Your ideal weight goes in the bottom space at the left, then number up to your present weight.

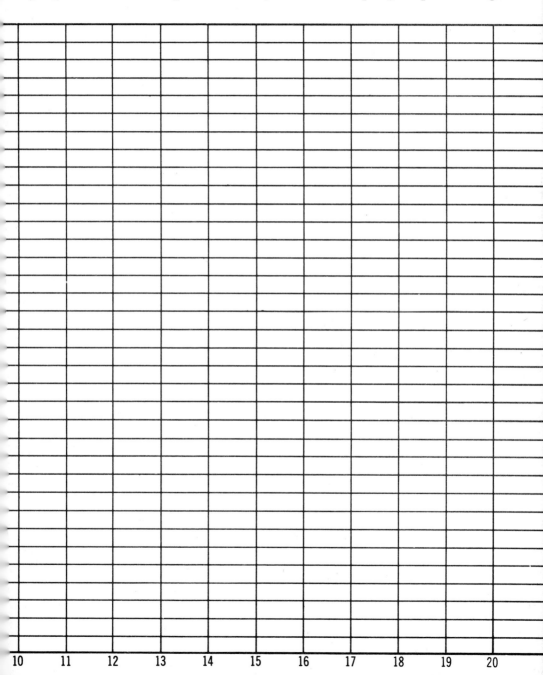

10   11   12   13   14   15   16   17   18   19   20